How to

Lose Your

Mother

Molly Jong-Fast

How to Lose Your Mother

A Daughter's Memoir

Picador

First published 2025 by Viking
an imprint of Penguin Random House LLC

First published in the UK 2025 by Picador
an imprint of Pan Macmillan
The Smithson, 6 Briset Street, London EC1M 5NR
EU representative: Macmillan Publishers Ireland Limited, 1st Floor,
The Liffey Trust Centre, 117–126 Sheriff Street Upper,
Dublin 1, D01 YC43
Associated companies throughout the world
www.panmacmillan.com

ISBN 978-1-0350-2933-4 HB
ISBN 978-1-0350-2934-1 TPB

Copyright © Molly Jong-Fast 2025

The right of Molly Jong-Fast to be identified as the
author of this work has been asserted by her in accordance
with the Copyright, Designs and Patents Act 1988.

All rights reserved. No part of this publication may be reproduced,
stored in a retrieval system, or transmitted, in any form, or by any means
(electronic, mechanical, photocopying, recording or otherwise)
without the prior written permission of the publisher.

Pan Macmillan does not have any control over, or any responsibility for,
any author or third-party websites referred to in or on this book.

1 3 5 7 9 8 6 4 2

A CIP catalogue record for this book is available from the British
Library.

Printed and bound by CPI Group (UK) Ltd, Croydon, CR0 4YY

This book is sold subject to the condition that it shall not, by way of
trade or otherwise, be lent, hired out, or otherwise circulated without
the publisher's prior consent in any form of binding or cover other than
that in which it is published and without a similar condition including
this condition being imposed on the subsequent purchaser.

Visit **www.picador.com** to read more about all our books
and to buy them. You will also find features, author interviews and
news of any author events, and you can sign up for e-newsletters
so that you're always first to hear about our new releases.

For my husband, Matt Greenfield

> Celebrity is the mask that eats the face
> of the wearer.
>
> John Updike

> I'd like to thank my terrible childhood
> and the Academy, in that order.
>
> Robert Downey Jr.

> I should note that the only advantage for a child
> in having an alcoholic parent is that you acquire,
> prematurely, quite a bit of valuable data.
>
> Gore Vidal

Prologue

I am the only child of a once-famous woman. How famous she was in her heyday I would argue is actually kind of irrelevant. Fame, like alcoholism, rings a bell in you that can never be unrung. My mother was famous, and changed the makeup of her cells like a smoker who gets lung cancer, or an addict who gets so hooked on heroin that she is never freed and has to go on methadone forever and ever—even after she's forgotten what the high of heroin was.

To say my mother and I are close doesn't really express the full magnitude of the relationship. We are painfully, inexorably, chronically close, the way magnets are. I'm not even sure sometimes in the night when I lie in bed staring at the ceiling that I exist without her to stick to. She created me and I enabled her. But there is a paradox at the heart of our relationship. As close as we were—are—there has always been, between us, an unbridgeable distance. My relationship with her has always been wildly conflicted. I know that she loved me. But I also know that she never really seemed particularly interested in me. She always told me she wanted me, desperately wanted me. But I spent most of my school breaks in a trailer park in Tampa with my nanny.

And as much as I love my mother, I've often found myself regarding her with feelings that are somewhat closer to the opposite of love. My relationship with her is split right down the middle. I admire her, but I pity her. I revere her—no, I *worship* her—but I am mortified by her. I'd always thought that there would be a time when I would finally be able to reconcile all these insane contradictory feelings, but not long ago, my mom started disappearing, began dissolving into the whiteness of the background, like a line on a shaken Etch A Sketch.

Now I have to write an obnoxious paragraph where I brag about who my mother is, or was. My mother is the writer Erica Jong. She is a novelist, essayist, and poet. She has published twenty-seven books, the most famous of which is her autobiographical novel *Fear of Flying*. It came out in 1973, five years before I was born, and is considered, in some corners at least, a landmark of feminist literature. Its candid depiction of women's sexual desires was extremely shocking at the time. It has sold over twenty million copies, and John Updike compared it to *The Catcher in the Rye* and *Portnoy's Complaint*. She created terms that are still part of our language. *Fear of Flying* made her very famous, for a writer. She was a guest on *The Tonight Show Starring Johnny Carson*. She was on the cover of *Newsweek*. Gore Vidal and Henry Miller were friends. I'm not here to brag about my mother's friendships with dead writers. But a lot of younger people have no idea who she is.

My mother coined an expression for casual sex: the "Zipless fuck."

Now think about being the offspring of the person who wrote that sentence. And pour one out for me.

I grew up with her everywhere—on television, in the crossword puzzle, in the newspaper. Mom was a kind of second-wave feminist, a white feminist, and an (highly educated, wildly affluent,

Jewish, and somewhat out-of-touch) everywoman. But she wasn't an actual everywoman, of course; she was too famous for that. Too famous, and too special. She was famous for that book, and then later she was famous for being famous, and then eventually she wasn't famous anymore. Because fame, like youth, is fleeting, it deserts you when you least expect it. The wheel of fortune is always spinning.

My mother never got over being famous. Even years after people stopped coming up to us in stores, even years after she slipped from the public consciousness, the virus of fame had already made her someone different. Becoming normal like the rest of us, the journey to unfamousness, was for her an event so strange and stressful, so damaging to her ego, that she was never able to process it.

My grandfather, the writer (and Communist) Howard Fast—his most famous novel was *Spartacus*, adapted into an even more famous movie directed by Stanley Kubrick and starring my grandfather's nemesis Kirk Douglas—had the curse, too: he was unable to become unfamous, to slip back into the world the rest of us occupy, the world of emptying the dishwasher and picking up your prescriptions, and the world of not having people stop you on the street to tell you every detail of their lives. My grandfather was a bestselling author who published over eighty books, but now no one—other than a very narrow subset of the elderly—has heard of him. I never knew my mother or grandfather in the height of their respective fames, but I did know them at the end, when they were desperately trying to claw fame back from the writers who, they believed, had taken it from them. Watching my mother's failed metamorphosis back to normal made me a sort of fame hobbyist, like a bird-watcher without the birds.

For the addictive personality, the junkie-itch from coming off celebrity can never ever be cured, not with all the adoration in the world. Mom was never a normal person again. My stepfather tried to keep her in the style to which she was accustomed, tried to treat her like a queen. Maybe it worked? I don't know. I never knew her when she was unfamous. She would always say that I was everything to her. She would always tell anyone who listened that I was her greatest accomplishment in life. I always knew that wasn't the truth.

I wondered if other people had the same connection issue with her that I did. I found her distracted and disinterested. Impossible to connect with. I always just assumed this was some personal failing on my part, just assumed the problem was me, but maybe other people felt the same way—they also assumed they were the problem. It would have been helpful to have a sibling to commiserate with, but I was my mother's only child. Everyone told me she loved me so much, but I never felt all that loved. Later on, I realized that I never felt that *anyone* loved me.

The pandemic broke my mom. When it started, she was her normal alcoholic self, not a hundred percent but she would do things and go places. By the end she was lying in bed all day drinking a bottle or two of wine. My stepfather was taking care of her, but he couldn't walk and was incontinent. They had a housekeeper who couldn't really help them, there were aides, but they were over their heads. I kept trying to help but they wouldn't let me. At some point I realized this was all my responsibility, at some point I realized that my mother had devolved into someone who was no longer in there. At some point I realized I was going to have to move them out of their house into a place. At some point, I found poop in my mom's bed. At some point I realized that the center would not hold. At some point I knew I had to intervene.

It was like the Yeats poem:

> Turning and turning in the widening gyre
> The falcon cannot hear the falconer;
> Things fall apart; the centre cannot hold;
> Mere anarchy is loosed upon the world,
> The blood-dimmed tide is loosed, and everywhere
> The ceremony of innocence is drowned;
> The best lack all conviction, while the worst
> Are full of passionate intensity.

I have always lacked all conviction; it wasn't until my forties that it occurred to me that I could possibly be right about things. Does this make me one of the best? Probably not, but it spared me from being one of the worst.

So it was the poop in the bed that made me know it was time. It was the poop in the bed that convinced me.

My mother is just a body now. She has dementia. She has breath and hair and pretty blue eyes but Erica Jong the person has left the planet.

My grandmother, my mother's mother, also had dementia and died at the exceptionally advanced age of a hundred plus, running through her money with a nurse who she thought was some kind of family member or friend. But that nurse had her own family.

I wasn't good about visiting Grandma. I was one of nine grandchildren and I used that as an excuse—diffusing the responsibility—but the truth was I just hated the idea of my grandma sitting in that bed, in a state between living and dead. Or maybe I was just a bad, selfish person? Or maybe I just didn't like old people, the reminder that death was around the corner, inching toward us. Grandma died, then Mom will die, and then I will. That's the best-case scenario. The worst-case scenario is that these things are out of order.

Like my grandmother, my mother will likely continue on for the next twenty-five years in a state of dreamy, distracted unreality. She will become increasingly unreachable. I recently gave an interview to NPR about my mother. The interviewer and I spoke in that weird, slightly halting NPR way. I kept flipping from the current to the past tense: "she was"; "she *is*." I couldn't quite agree with myself about if she was still on this planet or already gone.

I was a bad daughter. I am a bad daughter.

The horrible irony is that she has always seemed a bit demented. Maybe not demented, exactly, but distracted: dreamy, head-in-the-clouds, and detached. When I was a little red-haired girl—like Little Orphan Annie, but fat—I would yell at my mother for "spacing out." I used to beg her to focus, to pay attention to me. "Where did you go?" I'd ask her as she stared into space. My mother has these very glassy blue eyes. I would look into them and wonder if she saw me at all. Sometimes I'd wonder if I was real. Years later I would interview a journalist about Elon Musk and the journalist would tell me that there was evidence to support the supposition that Elon Musk believed he was in a simulation. The journalist continued, "A lot of rich and famous people believe that the world is a simulation for their benefit, because otherwise how could things have worked out so well for them?"

HOW TO LOSE YOUR MOTHER

I've been thinking a lot about this idea, that the entire world is just a simulation for your benefit.

Eventually, Mom would answer, but never the question I asked. She always seemed to have a sort of stock answer for even my stupidest, simplest questions, as if she were following her own script. She was always performing. Her father was a performer, too—a drummer in the Catskills before he became an importer, before he started his company, the Seymour Mann Connoisseur Collection, and sold his collectible dolls on QVC. (About him, my mother said in an interview with Charlie Rose, "He had put all of his vaudeville ambitions into me.") She would run her fingers through my hair and ask me if I knew how much she loved me. Did I know how much she loved me? Did I know how brilliant I was? How talented?

I wish I'd asked her why, if she loved me so much, she didn't ever want to spend time with me, but there was no way she'd have ever given me a straight answer. And besides, in her view, she *did* spend time with me—in her head, in her writing, in the world she inhabited. I *was* there. I may have felt that she was slightly allergic to me, but to her, she was spending time with the most important version of me.

Disassociation has always been her magic trick, her way of remaining in the world but also not. Was it her chronic dreaminess that made it impossible to tell if she was merely distracted, or if she was disappearing?

I'd always hated the idea of writing a book like this. I've always hated the idea that the luck of being born into a famous (ish) literary family might undermine anything else I've achieved. But this turns out not to be that story. This is the story of what happens when the bottom falls out, when all the tests come back bad, when the doctors tell you there's nothing more they can do. This is the story of the worst year of my life.

I've always been very conflicted about all of it, this book you're reading, these parents I have, or had, depending on how you see it. I'd written one very autobiographical novel, and then another less autobiographical novel, and I was bored with telling people about my life. Why would anyone care? *I* didn't even really care. I've made a career for myself as a political writer, and I can say that writing and thinking about politics has been a liberation for me. I don't *have* to write about myself or the people around me anymore. I grew up being written about. I know how annoying it is. Also, politics is horrible and fascinating, and my life is largely harmonious, and very dull. Or at least it was.

But I'm a writer, for better or worse. This is what I do. Yes, just like my mother. And it is my job to make sense of the past, of her life, of our relationship. My mother was unattainable, but I tried. I keep trying. Now she is slipping away and our story really is over. Just in time to try and make sense of it. I wrote this book to help people (you have to say that, but it's actually true), but also because I hoped the act of writing would make me less insane. No, not even insane—just less stuck. When I got sober, I was promised that I'd be able to see how my experience could benefit others. I truly believe this. So this is that.

Sometimes when I was working on this book, I bristled at the whole project of this memoir: a daughter trying to come to terms with the loss of a mother. But I never had Erica Jong. How can you lose something you never had?

1

For my entire life, random people have come over to "talk" to me about my mom. They wanted me to know how much they loved *Fear of Flying*. They wanted me to know how important her work was to them. They wanted to talk about her fame, about her inflammatory comments about sex. Sometimes they'd tell me some embarrassing thing she'd said about me on television. Sometimes they'd tell me about some embarrassing thing she'd written about me. But, starting four years ago, when I was writing for *The Daily Beast* and obsessed with tweeting, things started to change.

People were no longer coming up to me to tell me they had seen her on Charlie Rose or *Good Morning America*. (And Charlie Rose didn't have a show anymore; he'd been canceled.) Now people were coming up to me for a different reason, for one of those hard conversations. They would seem almost apologetic. They would pause before they spoke, their voices heavy with a kind of shame, a deep kind of embarrassment. It's always been hard for me not to find the discomfort of others deeply unpleasant. I'd encourage them to say whatever it was they wanted to—but did I want to hear it?

Their voices would inevitably be hushed and perhaps a bit halting. Sometimes the person would take my hand.

"How is your mother?" they would ask.

And then they would offer up one of the following comments:

"Is your mom . . . okay?"

"Are you *sure* she's okay?"

"She seems off."

"She can't remember anything."

"There's something really wrong with her."

Everywhere I went in my little neighborhood, I found myself surrounded by people who wanted to talk to me about my mother's failing memory and her increasingly erratic behavior: at the bookstore, at the hair salon, on the corner. Everywhere I went, my mother's condition followed me.

I went to a British restaurant for dinner with my husband and a famous poet—which is kind of an oxymoron, I know—and the poet's wife, a novelist. At the end of the dinner, the wife told me she had something to say that might upset me.

"No, it's okay," I said.

Was it okay? Who knows. I've always floated around like some kind of Erica Jong Rorschach test. I am a repository for people's feelings about my mother, about feminism, about the sexual revolution.

And then of course there is the little issue that my mother has never had a filter. She'd always say the worst possible thing. That was one of her trademarks. Sometimes when I'd be sitting at a dinner, or watching her give a talk, a thought would pop into my mind: "What is the worst possible thing she could say?" And, without fail, she'd say it. I remember watching in horror as someone live-tweeted her appearance at a book festival. I couldn't control what she said, or what people thought about her, but at least

HOW TO LOSE YOUR MOTHER

I could control one thing: when I was young, I decided not to read her books.

I braced myself for whatever the woman was going to say.

She explained that she had posted a photograph of her deceased father on Instagram. She picked up her phone to show me the post. I considered the picture of the woman's father. He looked like all deceased fathers: old.

"Your mother posted a comment on the photo," she said.

"Okay."

I was so past feeling embarrassed by things my mother said and did. I lived in this kind of perpetual post-embarrassment state. I could take this.

"The comment your mother wrote was 'Neat.'"

The woman looked as if she were going to cry.

I thought about my mother commenting on a picture of someone's dead father with the word "neat." And then it became difficult for me to think about much of anything else.

I called my stepfather, Ken. He had been a divorce lawyer. He was always ready to have a disagreement—not a fight exactly, but a sort of conflict, the kind I always hated.

"Hi, Ken," I said.

"Moll," he replied.

He always called me Moll.

"We have to talk about Mom."

He laughed. It was a pained laugh, an uncomfortable laugh.

"Mom is acting strangely," I said.

Ken cleared his throat.

"Mom is losing her memory," I said.

I could hear my mother's two poodles barking in their

apartment. I've known Ken since I was eleven years old. I knew the throat-clearing meant that he was getting prepared to lecture me about the thing everyone was telling me was true. Ken was one of those people who became a lawyer because he liked to fight, and he fought with anyone he could find. One of my more crushing childhood memories occurred when he yelled at a waiter because the restaurant didn't have his preferred mustard brand. He gave the waiter a twenty to go to the nearest deli and buy his stupid mustard. The waiter actually did it. That's how terrifying Ken was, but he could also be very kind. He often did my friends' divorces and undercharged them, or didn't charge them at all. He was never cruel to me. I did, however, feel that he believed he was put on this earth to protect my mother from me.

"Look, Moll, this is a hearing problem," Ken said. I had spent so many years arguing with him about what reality was and what reality wasn't, and each time he would tell me my reality was wrong and his was right. I hated arguing. I hated it. "She just needs hearing aids."

"*Ken*," I said. "This has nothing to do with hearing. She has dementia."

"Ah, Moll," he said. "You know she's just thinking of her next book."

But Mom hadn't written a book in a long time. The last thing she'd published was a book of poetry with a publisher that seemed like a vanity press. They had asked her for a donation. I'm not an economist or anything, but I think the publisher is supposed to pay the author.

And suddenly I was thirteen again, begging my stepfather to get my mother to stop taking diet pills, or to have her slow down on the drinking. Everyone told me I was crazy in that case, too. They would tell me that my mom she didn't drink too much; she was just tired. She was just passed out on the bed, eye makeup smeared all over her face, lipstick everywhere. She was just working on another book. She was just under a lot of pressure. Ken would inevitably declare, "Once she gets her book done then she'll be back to normal." Thirty years later, and I was having the exact same conversation with him. But this time, at forty-four, I finally knew my reality was right and his was wrong.

There was no book. There would never be another book. Her last tycoon, her swan song, was to be an autobiography called *Selfie*. She had gotten the idea that *Selfie* was a good title because, at a memorial service for a friend, she had run into David Remnick, the editor in chief of *The New Yorker*. She had told Remnick the title and she had decided he had liked it. It was not completely clear if this had actually happened, or happened in the way my mom was reporting it, but it didn't matter. That was her version of the story. It was always her version of the story.

"I think she's fine," Ken said calmly.

One of the interesting things was that you could say anything to my mom and stepdad, like *anything*, and they wouldn't get mad at you. Ken did love fighting, but part of the reason he loved it was because he never got really angry.

I told him that this was bordering on insane. I told him that everyone could see what was happening here.

"She wrote 'neat' on someone's Instagram post about her dead father. Like, 'Gee whiz, that's so neat that your father died.'"

"Eh," Ken said.

That was one of the many baffling things about both of them—when presented with evidence that perhaps they were wrong, they would just ignore the evidence and continue on their merry way. This habit of theirs always made me feel insane.

Ken was starting to display early symptoms of Parkinson's disease. He was in denial about that, too. One big difference between Mom and Ken: when Ken started losing his mind, he knew it. About ten years ago, he had told us. He wanted us to know, because he had a job, which was nominally still being a lawyer, but was really taking care of my mother. He was in his seventies when he started forgetting. Found himself to be less sharp. He started going to doctors. Doctors told him he was fine, but he knew. Soon after, he was diagnosed with Parkinson's. Then he sort of forgot about the anxiety that he was losing his mind and devoted himself to ignoring his Parkinson's.

This tactic was a stark contrast to my mom, who was now unable to remember if she'd fed the dogs or if she'd had a phone call. Everyone who talked to Mom knew that there was something deeply wrong with her. I don't know how many people suspected dementia. Given her dreamy nature, she had never seemed sharp per se, but—slowly, and then all of a sudden—she seemed completely lost. When confronted with this obvious fact, she would cover herself. She had many strategies. I'd misheard her; I had misunderstood her. She'd repeat a story she'd told me five minutes before, and I'd say, "You already told me this, Mom." Her response might be a defensive "I *know*"—as if the problem were mine for not appreciating that this story was important enough for her to keep repeating. Or she might try to change the subject by distracting me. Or she might just space out. She had a whole bag of tricks.

I texted my cousin Harold, who's a doctor. I wanted to know what the symptoms of dementia were. He texted back:

> Repetitive questions of things discussed and answered
>
> Short term memory loss
>
> Lack any deep thought and therefore quality of conversations diminished
>
> Facts that were shared on events etc became forgotten

Well, there you go. Check, check, check, check. Confirmed.

One evening a couple months later, I understood that her awareness of her condition had changed. She was sitting at the dining room table, drinking coffee and reading the paper when I came in the room.

"Hey," I said.

"Hi, darling."

She got up. Her silk robe was open and you could see her naked body. (She was never good at keeping her robe closed—this was true both metaphorically and literally.) She hugged me, she kissed me, she told me she loved me in an effusive way that was clearly not the way her own cold mean mom did it.

We sat down at the dining room table. I tried not to look at her boob, which was unfortunately somewhat visible. I spent way too much time thinking about getting older and about how ruthless the march of time was on the body.

I asked her if she wanted a cappuccino. She said she was okay.

"Mom, guess what?" I asked. "I saw your friend Judy at an event."

I'd just run into her old pal, the folk singer Judy Collins. Judy looked great—very thin and elegant, and dressed all in black.

She smelled great, too. Judy asked me how my mom was, because everyone always asked me how my mom was. I did not want to lie to Judy about my mother's increasingly demented condition, so I just made a face and said, "Meh."

"*Who?*" Mom asked.

"Your friend Judy. The *singer?*"

There was a faraway look in her eyes.

"Judy," she said. "Judy?"

I reminded her that she made Judy sing the Joni Mitchell song "Both Sides, Now" at my wedding. (Judy Collins had a hit with it in 1968.)

"*Judy!*" Mom declared. "Of course."

But I could tell she was lying. She had no clue who "Judy" was. Her voice always changed when she lied, became just the slightest bit more tentative.

And then she said, "I don't remember who that is."

That was the moment I realized she knew she couldn't cover anymore. She still wouldn't admit that she had dementia, but she would now occasionally admit that her memory wasn't what it used to be.

And then she kept slipping away—less and less of her in my life, less and less of her on the page, less and less of *her*. Soon she would be just a faint fragment of a once-great woman. She had been a force, a powerhouse, and now she was becoming an echo.

But it's very important for you to understand that Mom is one of those people who is constitutionally incapable of being honest. (She's been in denial about her drinking since I was born, for example.) Mom couldn't accept that she had dementia until she was so far gone it was no longer a question. But even then, she remained not convinced. Neither did Ken.

"Well, we just don't agree," Ken told me on the phone.

"She's going to Dr. Devi," I said. "I'm taking her to the dementia doctor."

Friends told me that Dr. Devi was one of the best neurologists in the city. I decided that she was going to save my mother. I'd heard stories about people who'd had their dementia paused by doctors, but I already worried that these people weren't like my mother. They were people who went to family reunions and didn't get DUIs. They were people who didn't get deeply drunk and give twenty-five-minute toasts for brides they never met at weddings they were barely invited to.

Dr. Devi was a beautiful woman who wore long, exotic-looking caftans and the Van Cleef & Arpels clover pendants I'd seen on the very fancy girls I grew up with. She had two gorgeous ancient rescue dogs in her office on Seventy-Sixth Street. She ran tests on my mother. She asked my mother some questions. Some of the questions were easy and some were harder. Some my mom could answer, but there were a lot she couldn't. I sat on the sofa and watched my mother try to remember the year she was born.

I've always had a kind of scrambled brain because of my dyslexia, so I weirdly related to my mother's half-cooked dementia-brain. Word retrieval has always been a problem for me. Names have caused me problems; words have never looked right. I sometimes think about how much easier life would be if I had one of those normal brains, one that just worked the right way.

Outside the window we looked out into a little courtyard. *This is it*, I thought to myself. *This is the moment it ends. This is the end of my relationship with my mom. The relationship I never got is over.*

The window is closing. Or it's closed. I will never get her attention now that the window is closed.

"Nineteen forty-two!" my mom answered with triumph.

Mom was right. She *was* born in 1942.

We all regarded this as a towering victory, like the defeat of the Athenians at Syracuse or Joan of Arc's conquest over the English.

We left the office and Mom and I stood together on Seventy-Sixth Street. It was a beautiful day in early September. I wore a light jacket. I wanted to enjoy these last minutes with her, but I had a piece due, a college essay to supervise. It was that super-subversive "Cat's in the Cradle" shit. She'd had her chance, and now I was busy. What can I say? I had to get stuff done. I didn't have time. She had missed my entire childhood, and I refused to miss my kids' childhoods for her.

I was so petty, even here, even at the end I was petty.

"Can you get home on your own?" I asked.

We were seven blocks from her building.

"*Of course* I can get home," she snapped. "Stop treating me as if there's something wrong with me."

I pointed her in the right direction. She looked tentative.

Another day of pretending, pretending she was okay, pretending she could get home alone. I was pretty sure she could get home, but not one hundred percent. I probably should have walked her home but I couldn't spare the time. I was suddenly seized with the image of my mother wandering the streets with no shoes. What if she got lost? What if I was doing to her what she'd done to me so many times: abandoning her? I thought about my normal life a few blocks uptown. I had worked so hard to pick up the glass shards of my childhood. I had put those shards back together and into something that vaguely resembled a life. I couldn't lose the life I had built now for my mother.

Mom still had a few friends, but she always had trouble getting along with people who were not men she wanted to seduce. (I probably shouldn't say that, but it's true.) She was one of those women who related best to men. Also, she had a pathological need to write about everyone all the time. Writing about people tends to infuriate them. I'd heard that Judy Collins was not at all happy because she apparently believed the protagonist of my mom's novel *Any Woman's Blues* was based on her. Sure, Leila Sand had gotten sober just like Judy Collins had gotten sober. And sure, Leila Sand was a folk singer, but Leila Sand was mostly Erica Jong. It was the *supporting* characters who were usually real people. I'd thought about explaining that to Judy, but I was already such a weird caretaker / supporting character in my own life, and I didn't know if I had the authority to tell Judy Collins anything.

My mother's staggering lack of self-awareness was what caused her the most problems. When I was in my twenties, there was an annual Valentine's Day lunch at the home of Judy Licht, a writer and local newscaster. Mom went every year. Sometimes she dragged me along. I watched as my mother delivered a kind of Oscar-style acceptance speech about her career and its many successes. The other attendees were ladies in their sixties, seventies, or eighties (I enjoyed being the youngest person in the room by at least thirty years), and they were all quite a lot better behaved than my mom. Dr. Ruth sat quietly and politely, even though she looked as if she wanted to throttle something or someone. Nora Ephron rolled her eyes. Nora was my mother's cooler peer, someone who seemed to have a real life with real friends and real relationships. My mom didn't have that. The grim embarrassment of this particular afternoon is still seared into my brain. I would have rolled my eyes if I could have. But I couldn't, of course, and I had to sit there like the good daughter I was. I was part of the problem. I was always part of the problem. I was the hostage-taker's plus-one. And so not only was Nora Ephron rolling her eyes at my mom, but she was also rolling her eyes *at me*. How many bad decisions did it take to end up in a position like this?

But the thing that made it just like every anxiety dream I've ever had was that there was nothing I could do to stop it. I just had to sit there wishing I was a fork.

The other problem with my mother is, well, the *drinking*. She is one of those "high-functioning" alcoholics. This fact is highly debated in my family. Maybe there are families where people admit their loved one is an alcoholic. This was not my family. Even at the end, even when my grandmother was drinking herself into oblivion, even then no one ever wanted to admit that Grandma was an alcoholic. "She doesn't really drink anymore" was the refrain offered, but she'd been an alcoholic and her alcoholism had rippled through all our lives like a flesh-eating virus. Excuses were made, as they always are. She had Crohn's disease. She was sick. She was upset about Grandpa dying. No one ever wants to say anyone is an alcoholic. Alcoholism continues to feel like a moral failing as opposed to a genetic abnormality. There's always a sense that maybe if the alcoholic could just work a little harder maybe they could just get it under control. But when the alcoholic is "high-functioning," or famous, or was famous, it's even harder for the family to help them.

I always tell people I'm sober because I feel as if I'm in a position to destigmatize the disease, to show people you can get sober as a teenager and stay sober. But a lot of the time people believe that because I'm sober, I automatically think everyone is an alcoholic. I don't, but I do think everyone in my *family* is an alcoholic.

Here is a recurring event from both from my childhood and from later in my adulthood: my mother weeping in her chair, apologizing to me for being an alcoholic. "I'm sorry, darling. I'm sorry." And in that moment, she always was.

In her clearer moments my mom would tell me she was an alcoholic, and she would then hold forth about my grandmother's alcoholism. Grandma's being a drunk was something we sort of talked about. Grandma Eda got drunk at all family events until she got very, very old. Before that, she would get drunk and vomit at all the best Manhattan restaurants. "Grandma is a drunk but so am I," my mother would say, shamefully.

But about an hour later, she'd be enjoying her huge glass of white wine.

An important caveat is that my mother wasn't a mean alcoholic like my grandmother (who used to get drunk, and scream at everyone, and pull off her clothes on the crosstown bus). But Mom wasn't *in there* when she drank, even when she *was* in there. My mother wasn't bad, she was just gone.

I got sober in Hazelden in Center City, Minnesota. I remember my last drink like it wasn't twenty-five years ago: three vodka cranberries in the lounge, two Klonopin, and then three glasses of white wine on the plane. My mom flew with me, but she left me in the Minneapolis airport with the little old lady who drove me in her station wagon to the rehab center. Mom turned around and flew home, back to cocktail parties and her normal late-nineties New York City life. I often wonder if my mom drank on the flight home. I would have. I absolutely would have.

Mom went back to Dr. Devi for some more tests. A week later, she and I were supposed to go back to the office for the results.

She canceled that appointment. She told me Dr. Devi said she was fine, that she didn't really have dementia. I think I knew she was lying when she told me, but I wanted to believe the lie. The truth sucked too much. Ken decided that Dr. Devi was wrong. Mom agreed. My poor disoriented mother was trying to remember if she fed the dogs, but clearly, she didn't have dementia. What did the doctors know anyway? They were just doctors. That powerful denial that helped Ken deal with Mom's drinking, the denial that had helped him for so long in work, life, and love, was keeping him from acknowledging the truth. I might say something here about how they both gaslit me, but gaslighting implies they had some belief in the truth, and I don't think they did. Both my mother and stepfather occupied the same nonexistent world. They had their truth, which I do believe they thought in their hearts was *the* truth.

But here's the thing . . . the truth didn't matter. There is no cure for dementia. There is no treatment. There is nothing to do but sit there and watch the person you love disappear. So maybe his denial once again helped him. Maybe *I* was the stupid one.

But you can't be fine from dementia. It's not over just because you say it's over.

This is where I need to reiterate that my mother has always been almost entirely without self-reflection. She can't ever look back at something and take stock of it. It has always been too painful for her to pause and wonder if perhaps she could have done things differently. Not being able to learn from past mistakes makes any kind of forward progress almost impossible. As a sober, I spend a lot of time thinking about the possibility of learning from mistakes. It was entirely in keeping with my mother's character that she was unable to acknowledge this final, devastating truth about herself.

One afternoon several days later, Dr. Devi called me out of the blue. I had just landed in DC for a twenty-four-hour visit. I was in a red taxi, wearing a mask. I didn't want to take the call, but I knew I had to.

"Mom said you gave her a very optimistic diagnosis," I said, trying to sound as cheerful as possible.

"That's absolutely *not* what I told her," Dr. Devi said.

For a moment, I was seized by rage. There were mothers who didn't always lie to their children. There was a normal world out there filled with normal people who weren't sociopaths, and none of them would ever be my mother.

"At best, your mother has dementia," she said. "At worst, Alzheimer's."

"Oh," I said.

I wanted to say something else. I wanted to tell the doctor the bigger truth and explain that I'd never known her, that she'd never known me. That I loved her, that I burned for her, but that none of it was enough. How could I say that? You can never tell anyone the whole truth. As the daughter of Erica Jong, I'd gotten pretty good at whitewashing reality.

I ended the call and felt something that's very hard to describe. It was the bereft, broken feeling of something ending before it ever got the chance to start.

I checked into my hotel. I did some work. I ate a candy bar from the minibar. I decided that I had to call my stepfather. I hated being my parent's parent, and I had done mountains of cocaine and had drunk myself to oblivion to free myself of this role.

Hadn't worked. I should have known that sooner or later we all become who our parents make us.

Ken picked up the phone.

I heard myself saying the astonishing words, "Mom has dementia. Or maybe Alzheimer's."

Silence from Ken, he knew I was right, but he couldn't say it, so he said nothing. The barking of their dogs.

Finally, Ken spoke.

"I'm going to let you talk to her," he said.

He spoke to her offstage. I could hear the muffled sounds of their voices.

And then my mother's voice, transmitted into the phone two hundred and fifty miles away.

"Hello?" she asked. The voice, so familiar to me, had a different character about it. She sounded hesitant . . . *frail* almost—two things my mother has never been.

"Dr. Devi called me, Mom," I said. "She told me you have dementia."

"Really? But I *do* remember *some* things?"

I thought about the things *I* remembered from my childhood, a scattered tapestry of hotel rooms, sitting alone at lunch tables praying no one would notice me. *We all remember some things*, I wanted to say. I wanted to tell her I remembered all the times she couldn't stand to be alone in a room with me and couldn't wait to flee to her office, or didn't take me on trips with her, but I'm forty-four years old and twenty-five years sober, and I'm too old and too sober to be an asshole to my aging mother, who tried her best with me, at least when she was aware of my existence.

"You have dementia," I said again.

HOW TO LOSE YOUR MOTHER

A heavy pause.

"I have . . . dementia?" she asked again.

"Yes, Mom," I said, "you do."

2

It was a week that felt like a year, one of those weeks that contained all the scary things you might spend your life worrying about, the things that might never happen. Our very elderly diabetic dog, Spartacus, had had a grand mal seizure on our bed. During the seizure, I wondered if I too had slipped into unreality. (That was the problem with the demented-mother thing: I was so codependent, so enmeshed, that I always wondered if I also had the same bad brain my mother did.) Spartacus bit his tongue and bled all over the fancy quilt I bought with the money from my podcast. Spartacus survived, continuing his existence as an animal now largely Scotch-taped together. The seizure occurred the night after Matt and I had signed the power of attorney for my eighty-one-year-old mother and eighty-two-year-old stepfather. Or maybe the seizure was the night after that? It was just too much to absorb between the dog and my mother and my stepfather. All these things happened during the same week, but the order of them was in my mind never entirely clear.

It had already been three years since we started talking about Mom's mind going. It had been almost two years since we'd gotten the diagnosis from Dr. Devi. Covid had finally gone away but you wouldn't have known it, since Mom and Ken never left the apartment. Ken had settled into Parkinson's. He refused to do much of the treatment plan. Mom could still remember who I was, but often not a lot else. Sometimes she didn't remember her grandchildren. Sometimes she didn't remember that she is—that she was—a writer. Things didn't fit together for her anymore. Sometimes she was a little girl, and sometimes her parents were still alive. She and Ken spent a lot of time in their living room, reading, or trying to read, the paper. The weird thing was that, although they had no idea what was going on, they actually seemed pretty happy. But I knew that they were at the end of the road, happiness-wise. I knew what was to come, and I feared it, and so with the lawyers I did the papers that would let me take over my parents' lives.

And then the writer Fay Weldon died. I didn't know Fay all that well, but I loved her. I'd stayed at her house a few different summers when I was a druggy teen in the nineties. She was the kind of writer I had always wanted to be. Hilarious, stylish, sardonic, and also just completely focused on the plight of the middle-aged woman. She was funny, but also had a rage that I admired. I had spent the day of Saturday, January 7, working on an essay about her. Even though she was ninety-one, I was bereft about her death. Because I'm a terrible person, Fay's death wasn't, for me, really about Fay; Fay's death was about the end of *my* life, my nineties life, that is, the end of summers smoking pot on Hampstead Heath. But the big trauma of a week of traumas was to come later that night.

Matt went to the ER that Saturday evening for stomach pains. He'd believed the irritation was caused by the weird diet drug he was taking, because it gave everyone diarrhea and bloating. It's a drug whose side effects basically mimic Crohn's disease, a disorder my family knows well, since one of our kids has been suffering from it since he was five. I went to bed, sad about Fay, sad about the dog, sad about my mother's future. But I wasn't worried about Matt. Yet.

I was sleeping, or sort of sleeping, when my phone rang at 3:00 a.m.

"They found a mass on my pancreas," Matt said.

I responded to Matt with one of the things people say when confronted with bad news. I can't remember the exact string of words. Maybe I said "Fuck." Maybe I said "No." Maybe I said something else, maybe I offered a platitude. I had gotten good at platitudes recently. I had gotten really good at talking but conveying very little actual content.

"They say they think it's maybe probably possibly cancer," he added. "I'm going to walk home."

That phrase "Maybe probably possibly cancer" jangled in my head. My husband comes from one of those cancer families—his aunts, uncles, and a cousin: all dead from cancer. Even though Matt and I are distantly related, my family isn't a cancer family like that. We're an autoimmune family: Crohn's (as I said), MS, Parkinson's—all the nasty stuff that doesn't kill you right away but that you suffer with for years, for decades and decades. Like being stuck sitting next to my mother when she makes one of her drunken toasts—the Jong brand is all about suffering.

An hour later, a half hour later, two hours later—who knows—Matt came home and got into bed. I stared at the wall and told him I didn't want him to die. Or maybe I dreamed that part. I was never a good sleeper as a child. I would sleepwalk. Sometimes I just wouldn't sleep for nights and nights in a row. I thought about the article I read about the Italian family of aristocrats who didn't sleep. They each went mad and died. I understood this now.

I have been with Matt since I was twenty-three. That's more than twenty years, for those doing the math. I've never been an adult without him.

I didn't sleep at all that night. All I could think about was the idea of living without him. Matt, I should add, is not one of those people who is easy to live with: he is removed, hard to connect with, sometimes fragile, and slightly terrified of people. I am not that way: I'm bossy and annoying. I'm just as hard to live with, but in an entirely different way. And of course, you don't marry someone who is fourteen years older than you are without the knowledge that you will probably outlive them, but I had never played it out like this. Matt was only fifty-nine.

The following morning was Sunday. We stared at each other blankly and tried to think of things to say that would stop us from feeling scared. What lie would we tell our children? Matt wanted to tell them the truth. I wanted to lie. Should we call it a "mass" or a "tumor"? We decided we didn't want to call it a tumor because a "tumor" sounded quite a lot scarier. A "mass" could be anything—a group of people, a group of blood vessels, a group of cockapoos meeting in Central Park for a cockapoo meetup.

We pretended to be normal people that day. We did things normal people do. I didn't visit my mother in the weird apartment that smelled like dog poop that I would soon need to move her out of. I couldn't handle the added stress of her weird state. Instead, I just watched *The Larry Sanders Show* with my eldest child, who was supposed to go back to college in a few days.

Later in the afternoon, Matt told me about all the places he'd stashed our money—in checking accounts and in crypto. He was oddly thrilled to tell me about all these contingency plans. When you've spent your entire life obsessing about worst-case scenarios, there's something weirdly gratifying when it happens. I didn't mention this to him, of course, but I couldn't help noticing that Matt had . . . well, a smell. It was a smell that showers seemed unable to dislodge. He smelled sick. I'm not a doctor (I mean, obviously), but I've always been able to tell when people are sick.

I kept having obsessive thoughts. I kept thinking, "I am a widow. I am a forty-four-year-old widow." But one of the benefits of being the daughter of a world-class narcissist is that I can look at my situation and know that I shouldn't behave in it the way my mother would. I kept thinking about when my stepfather was diagnosed with Parkinson's—it was before my mother was diagnosed with dementia and I could tell that she was actually toying with the idea of leaving him. I could tell it was happening right in front of my eyes. I could feel it. Even later on, as her memory started to go, she still experimented with the idea of putting him in a home.

I remember the following strange exchange like it was yesterday. We were sitting in her office, drinking coffee. She was speaking in hushed tones. I kept wondering what she was getting at. It's funny, but even after so many years of knowing my mother, I could still be surprised at who she was. Or maybe it was that I just could never really *accept* who she was.

"Maybe it's time to put your stepfather somewhere," she said. "Somewhere he can get the help he needs."

As soon as I realized what she was saying, I was furious with her. Yet I understood why she was saying it. He had stopped being able to devote himself to her. He had stopped being the person she had married. For so many years Mom had made me compete with Ken for her love, and now I had won—sort of. But I wasn't going to enable this betrayal.

"No, Mom. We're not doing that. You are not leaving Ken."

Here is something crucial to remember: I am the product of that person, that person who left every man the instant he got sick, or, even worse, boring. That woman created me.

A friend whose mom died of pancreatic cancer gave me the name of one of the best pancreatic cancer doctors in New York City, Dr. O'Reilly. Of course, being that it was pancreatic cancer, her mom died a few months after diagnosis, like most people with pancreatic cancer. The doctor said she could fit us in on Tuesday.

My college kid went back to school. I told him not to worry about his father. I told him that his dad had cancer but that he was going to be fine. The college kid didn't believe that his dad was going to be fine, but it didn't matter. We hugged, tacitly agreeing that he would believe my lie for now.

He's always been the most delicate of the children. He got into a car to the airport. It was raining. In my first novel, the novel I wrote about getting sober when I was a teenager, the main character (me) gets into a car in the rain to go to rehab. But my kids weren't fucked-up drug-addicted teens like I was. They were just normal people with normal lives, not obsessive addicts.

We read up on the cancer before the appointment. My friend sent me a list of questions for the doctor. In the list were hideous terms like "tumor sequencing." At once, I realized this was going to be the single thing in my life that eclipsed everything else, even more of a cataclysm than my mother's dementia. I didn't really have the time to have everything eclipsed; I had my columns to write, and people to interview for my podcast.

The tumor the ER doctors found was small—two centimeters—and located in a good part of the pancreas, in the tail. Easier to remove, a doctor friend told us. You really don't want it closer to the duct, which is apparently more vascular. (How I wish I did not now know these things. I don't want to know anything about pancreases. Or tails.)

Matt would go to Sloan Kettering, the fancy cancer hospital, the one that had the fancy parties. Matt would have the best fancy pancreas doctor. One look at Google, however, made it clear that a tumor on the pancreas was no one's idea of a happy ending.

I felt kind of sick. Matt was the sick one, but I felt as if I was going to die. That smell, that slightly sour smell, was still there, which also meant that Matt was going to die. I didn't want to say anything. I was sure of it, though. I was sure about what that smell meant.

Even in those moments, those hours of waiting for the doctor's appointment, and knowing so little, even then it was still less awful than the horrible powerlessness I felt growing up. Yes, it was lonely and sad. I was, however, an adult. No one was going to forget to pick me up at school. Matt could die, I didn't want him to, but it could happen and I could handle it. I would be devastated but I would be an adult, and not a child lost at an airport or a train station.

The day of Matt's first appointment came, and we took a taxi to Sloan Kettering, in an office building in Midtown. The waiting room was filled with very elderly gray-haired people. Matt was the youngest sick person there by several decades. I was seized by self-pity. I couldn't help it. We were in the middle of our lives not at the end. They had had their lives, we were just in the middle, we were supposed to have a few more decades of normal before arriving at this confrontation with the end.

It wasn't fair. Why our bad luck? Why? But self-pity was the worst thing we could do, the worst thing we could feel.

It was only about 4:00 p.m., but somehow it had gone from cloudy to almost black rather quickly, and I couldn't help but feel that the weather was for the first time accurately reflecting my mood. And my mother still had dementia, of course. Would any of these people in the waiting room want to trade places with my mom? Would you rather lose your mind, or die? Would you want to hold on, even if it meant that every day you became less yourself and more *someone else*? I couldn't think of my husband's illness without thinking of my mother. I could have used a little spacing out, honestly.

Dr. O'Reilly was small, blond, and Irish. My friend had already warned me that this doctor wasn't the warm and fuzzy type. These kinds of doctors never are.

Matt sat on the examination table. He looked like Eeyore. Given that all his aunts and uncles had died of cancer in their fifties, had he always thought this would happen to him, too? And had I? He had made it through his fifties without cancer—well, almost.

The unapproachable Irish doctor was giddy. The thing about doctors who specialize in diseases that kill seventy to eighty percent of their cases is that they are delighted to have a patient who might not necessarily die imminently.

"We think this surgery could be curative," she said.

We paused and looked at each other like people in a movie.

"You could be cured," she continued, in case we didn't understand her.

It was clear to me that this doctor didn't get to say these sorts of sentences very often.

Immediately, I had a kind of shift in my thinking. I don't know if I get these abrupt emotional shifts because I'm sober and have spent many hours in AA meetings, thinking about how adversity can be good for spiritual development, or if there's some other reason, but I tend to be able to see the good even in the bad. And for a minute, in that exam room in that weird and horrible Sloan Kettering Midtown office building, I felt exceedingly grateful. Sure, it was scary. Sure, Matt would have to go through some things. Sure, the children would need to be managed, lied to, whatever . . . but he wasn't going to die. Matt was one of the very few people who went into that office and weren't told they would die.

That word "curative." There was a cure. There might be a hard road for him and for us but there was a cure. He wouldn't die. He would be cured.

A week later, I went to a small dinner with a group of women in media. It was in the basement of a fancy restaurant, somewhere you couldn't get a reservation—you had to know someone or have a special fancy email address. The guests were very accomplished women. They went around the room and talked about their anxieties and their accomplishments. At some point, someone mentioned that I was writing a memoir about my mother's dementia. Everyone applauded. I cringed.

I felt like a total fraud. Maybe Mom *didn't* have dementia. Maybe she was just getting old. Maybe I was making the whole thing up. I was doing the thing my mother had done her whole life: making shit up.

HOW TO LOSE YOUR MOTHER

I've always said that I felt comfortable writing about my mother because she always wrote about me. I didn't feel comfortable in that moment, though, with this group of intimidating women applauding me for betraying my mother, my sick mother, my tragic subject-matter. My sick husband had also now become another bit of tragic subject-matter. A woman patted me on the shoulder and told me I was a good daughter. In what world does betraying your mother equal being a good daughter? But I wasn't just writing about her, I was writing about someone totally innocent. I was writing about my husband, who was sick. Was I also a bad spouse? Was I betraying Matt, too?

Yes, I was. I was a double-betrayer.

I was reminded of a Christmas when I was seventeen. It was snowy and I was driving from my mother's house in Weston, Connecticut, to my father's house in Cos Cob. My mother stopped me before I got into the car. She looked concerned. Had she been drinking? It was early in the morning so perhaps not, though not impossible, not impossible at all.

"Please be careful when you're driving," she said. She held my hand. "I don't want you to slide off the road and end up dead on Christmas."

"Mom, we're *Jewish*," I said and got into my black 1993 Saab. "The last time I checked, Jews don't celebrate Christmas." We did of course celebrate Christmas because we were assimilated.

Later, I would wonder if it was possible, maybe just a little bit possible, that my mother sort of *wanted* me to drive off the road. Of course, she loved me. I was her only child. But *life* was her only material. And bourgeois life is boring, filled with shopping trips and boring interactions with other boring affluent people. Rarely was there a tragedy in bourgeois life, so we always had to go and make our own. I often wondered if a small part of her hoped for this material. I wasn't a good driver, but I wasn't going to be someone else's tragedy. I was committed to being my *own* train wreck, not anyone else's, and certainly not my mother's.

Another thing that I want you to know about my mother is that she was a real celebrity to me. She was very glamorous. She had that weird magic famous people have, where you never know what other famous person they might be hanging out with, or what fabulous city they might be jetting off to. Mom had that fairy dust. You never knew who would be calling her on the phone. Once when I picked up the phone, Oprah was on the other end. There was just a feeling with Mom that anything could happen. Sometimes a limousine would show up outside the house and she'd be whisked away for days, or weeks. Sometimes my nanny and I would know where she was going, sometimes we would not. She was singularly the most glamorous and inaccessible person I'd ever known. She would often complain that she'd spent all the book money. She'd lie awake at night worrying about how we'd survive another month, how she'd be able to pay for my expensive private school. But then sometimes she'd take me out on extravagant shopping trips despite needing said cash. There was always a sense that reality and her actions weren't actually all that connected. The magic of fame made it very hard, almost impossible, for her to be a normal responsible person.

And greatly adding to her appeal was the fact that she was never ever free. A piece was due, a book needed to be written, a dinner party was being thrown in her honor, a new stepfather was just around the corner. A TV show needed her to speak on abortion rights, and the pill, and feminism. Sometimes I would go with her and sit in a greenroom that was almost never green and someone would offer me a cup of water and a cookie. Once a girl in a green room called me the "Jongette." I wondered why she didn't like me. She didn't even know me. If she knew me, she'd like me, I'd make sure of it.

I became good at getting people to like me, skilled. Did I like *them*? Didn't matter. What mattered was that *you* liked me, that you thought you wouldn't but then after a few minutes, found it was hard not to. It ended up being the most important skill: getting people to like me, winning them over. And did this rather manipulative tactic also work in my relationship with my mother? It did. Oh, yes, it did, because my mother *loved* me. My Jewish mother loved me the way Jewish mothers love their sons.

Sometimes I would wonder if the person had read my mom's books and knew something terrible about me, like how bratty I was, or that I couldn't read all throughout lower school, or how I was fat even as a toddler, or how I had had a terrible time learning my letters. So much of my shame was wrapped up in my learning disability. But more of my shame was wrapped up in not knowing what you'd read about me.

Now, somehow, the tables are turned and I'm doing to her exactly what she always did to me. Do I pretend that I am absolved—or at least safe in my public judgments about her—because I know she will never be able to read what I'm writing?

3

My parents met in California. They were introduced by my grandparents—Communist hero Howard Fast and his wife, Bette Fast, the daughter of newspaper-distribution man Ike Cohen. Both Howard and Bette and my mom had been friendly with an old poet named Louis Untermeyer who lived in Newtown, Connecticut. Grandpa said that he'd have a party for Mom when her latest book came out. The day of the party, the bartender—who was also to act as the evening's chauffeur—didn't show up, so Grandpa put my dad to work: he had to pick up my mom at her hotel.

My dad had a green MG. He had hair then. He, with his hair and his sporty little MG, met my mom at her hotel. A few weeks later, she was in the Dominican Republic, getting a divorce from her second husband, Dr. Allan Jong, the star (sadly for him) of *Fear of Flying*. My mom said that her divorce lawyer in Santo Domingo was also her taxi driver. After the divorce was finalized, her driver/attorney took her out for ice cream.

When my parents got together, my father's parents were living in a modest home behind the Beverly Hills Hotel. There were still modest homes in Beverly Hills back in the seventies—now there's an enormous five-story parking complex on the site.

HOW TO LOSE YOUR MOTHER

After they were married, my parents bought a house—a shack, really—on the wrong side of the Pacific Coast Highway, in Malibu. In the late nineties, my mom dragged me with her to go have a look at the house. It still had a spray-painted snake on the garage door. When they lived there, the neighbors on one side were a rock band; on the other was my mother's friend the writer Henry Miller. (My mother always insisted she never slept with him, but who knows.) That California, the California of the seventies, was a different world, a world filled with sprouts and yoga and lots of sweet sticky pot.

My mother and father were madly in love, or so they said. But it's possible that every parent tells their child that. Or put it another way, I don't think my mother was ever *not* madly in love.

After a couple of months, they moved back to the East Coast, because they were worried that having a child grow up on the West Coast would make said child weird and fucked up. Yes, the West Coast would fuck a kid up, but the decade over the course of which they spent divorcing soon after seemed not to bother them much at all.

New York City was considered dangerous back then, so my parents moved to Weston, Connecticut, a small town thirty minutes from the Merritt Parkway near New Canaan. Close to us was the home / animal shelter owned by the younger sister of Gypsy Rose Lee, June Havoc. (You will remember the character of Baby June from the musical *Gypsy*.) My parents adopted a dog from Gypsy Rose Lee's sister because of course they would adopt a dog from Gypsy Rose Lee's sister. I mean, why not? They named the dog Buffy. Buffy had red fur and was always sick and had all sorts of parasites. They also had a white bichon called Poochkin, who was unfortunately very stupid.

The house they bought was on a small patch of land and was constructed of old barns. There was an office for her and an office for him. My father was a writer, too. They would write all day, call each other on the intercom, eat organic food, smoke pot, get drunk, and irritate their neighbors. My father ate meat and smoked cigarettes. It's still hard to think about him as someone who had hair.

In August 1978, I was born in a hospital in Stamford, Connecticut. I came out with red hair. This was proof to my mother that I was special. The fantasy of my specialness continued my entire life. I was special even though I was dyslexic. I was special even though I got kicked out of Dalton. I was special even though I was a drug addict. I was special despite my fatness. I was special despite all the evidence to the contrary. I was special because I was a piece of her.

I read an interview with my mother in which the interviewer described me as a "stout" toddler. "Stout" means "kind of fat." I never thought of a toddler as being able to be fat, but there it was.

This is from that interview in *The Washington Post*: "Their daughter, Molly Miranda Jong-Fast, is 2 years old and red-headed. She was born between pages 284 and 285 of 'Fanny.' Having the baby, Jong says, 'transformed' her. 'In my 20s and early 30s I didn't think I wanted children,' she says. 'But by the time I was 34 or 35, I realized that if I didn't have a baby soon, it was going to be a matter of picking up every stray dog in Connecticut.'"

I always wondered if they would have been better off with a dog. Later, my mom bought a dog and named it the name she had wanted to name me, the name my father wouldn't let her use: Belinda.

The house was basically a 1970s time capsule. There were

levels in the attic and those levels were covered in a brown shag carpet. (That carpet was still in place when we finally sold the house during the real-estate mini-boom of the pandemic.) My parents slept in a waterbed. Outside was a big wooden hot tub and a sauna. The three of us lived there with my nurse, Lula, who, my mother said, based on no actual evidence, ran numbers for the Mafia out of nearby Bridgeport.

What happened, what ended the union, I never could get a straight answer about. There was definitely infidelity, much of it chronicled in my mother's writing. There was jealousy—or that was my mother's story. "Your father always thought he'd get famous too," she'd say. But fame isn't contagious. I don't actually believe my father was jealous of her success. What I do believe is that Mom quietly concocted the most hurtful way to put him down. Mom wasn't spiteful like my grandmother Eda was, but she was singularly brilliant at figuring out the weak spots, the places where the flesh was not supported by bone. This is what happens when you're raised by someone as cunning as my grandmother.

The reason I knew Mom was a liar was because her story always changed. Sometimes it was one thing, then sometimes it was an entirely different story. This shifting reality, this strange post-truth ecosystem she inhabited, and that I for a time inhabited too, made me completely unable to know what was real and what was a lie with her. It was a kind of gaslighting by proxy, like Munchausen syndrome, but somehow much, much stupider. I grew up with a lot of mistrust about people. I was prickly. I was hard to connect with. I didn't trust anyone. When I got sober at nineteen, I learned how to be an actual person. Before that I would do all sorts of alienating things and feel surprised when people felt alienated by me.

As I've gotten older, I've become more generous toward my fellow humans. I eventually learned that not everyone is a serial killer . . . or a serial fabulist.

Later my mother admitted they had an open marriage. My father, when questioned about this, said only, "Yes, she *thought* it was open."

"He was just too jealous of me," she would tell me. My father was, at the time, working toward a master's in social work. She said that kind of thing a lot, and about a lot of people. My father often said she was impossible to live with, an experience I've had firsthand. Should I blame the way she became on her fame, on all the years of people telling her she'd changed their lives? Or perhaps she was always like that.

By the time I was born, *Fear of Flying* was already five years old. My unfamous father married a very famous woman, though they actually didn't get married until my mom was pregnant with me because they both believed marriage was a bougie construct.

My father's famous father hadn't been jailed or blacklisted since the 1940s, but he was still famous—or notorious—sort of. And Grandpa ended up back on the *New York Times* bestseller list much later too, in the eighties, with a bunch of pulpy historical fiction novels. So my father had the double bad luck of being married to a famous writer and being the son of a famous writer.

Even back then, I think (though I don't know this firsthand, because I wasn't actually there) that Mom was anxious about losing her fame. Almost from the moment she got famous she was worried about becoming unfamous. The truth was that Mom never understood how she got famous, and never thought she deserved it. So I think that made her even more afraid that the condition was merely on loan.

But being a famous writer is not like being a Kardashian. It's not even like being a famous politician. First of all, being a famous writer means that people tend to know your name, but not necessarily your face. This fame usually peaks and ebbs, and the peaks occur with the publication of a book. I always knew there was something strange that united my grandfather and my mother, something that made them both so unbearable to deal with. I'm not sure I knew it was "fame"—that unmeasurable metric. I did know that my mom and my grandfather were always very busy. They were too busy to do the things that normal humans were expected to do.

My grandmother Bette did everything for my grandfather, like *everything*. They had someone who came in and cleaned, but Bette was Grandpa's liaison to the real world. I mean, except for his extracurricular activities (or affairs, I should say), which I assume he handled himself.

Mom clearly understood that fame was, even for most famous people, a temporary state. She was indeed always convinced that someone might try and take her career away; the problem was, she was pretty sure it was *me* who might take her career away. I think she truly believed that having kids killed my grandmother's career; it was one of those weird multigenerational lies that kept going on and on. But the truth was that alcoholism was much more of a career-killer for Grandma than having kids.

Eventually, my dad moved out of our house. It was one of those epic divorces with teams of lawyers. Maybe you've seen the movie *Irreconcilable Differences*? It was a bit like that except everyone was less attractive. And then my *mom* also moved out of the house! She left me in Weston with my nanny, Margaret. Mom moved to New York and did the very seventies thing of sharing an apartment with another single gal—the aforementioned Judy Licht. Let's politely call the place where they lived their bachelorette pad. I stayed in the house in Weston for a year with Margaret, and eventually we were summoned back to New York. My mom had met a guy named Cash. He was in his twenties, and handsome. I assumed he was dumb, maybe he wasn't. He was gone by the time I was old enough to make the assessment as to whether or not he was stupid. I know he desperately wanted to be an actor. Did he think Mom could make him famous? This was always a question I would ask myself: *If I were Mom, would I assume this person is using me?* Not sure Mom ascribed such cynical motives to people. I think she was more trusting than I am, perhaps even way too trusting. Despite having grown up in a seriously crazy family, Mom was never dark like I am. She had a sunny optimism that baffled me.

Mom kept the place in Weston as her country house. I grew to loathe that house. Mostly it was the association of being left there alone with Margaret that year. (Later, there was the problem of being dragged there every weekend only so I could watch my mother read the paper and my stepdad work on his legal cases.) I understand that being bored is not abuse, and during the eighties it was much more common to just have children and ignore them. This whole child-centered thing really didn't catch on until the nineties, as we know. By the time I had my kids we knew you were supposed to pay attention to them and honestly, I've been delighted to get to do it. My kids are the reason I'm on this planet, and raising them is the great joy of my life.

It's funny because when I was young my mom would tell me she was a great mom, then when I got a bit older, she would tell me that she practiced "benign neglect"—as if this parenting style was somehow by design.

One day after she had tried this line on me too many times (obviously she felt terrible about the sort of mother she was), I just snapped and said, "It was just *neglect* neglect. Benign makes it sound intentional. Stop *saying* that."

She never said it again.

I know how entitled I seem, complaining about my childhood. I mean, I never worked in a factory. I never ever wanted for one single material possession. Ever. Not once. I know how lucky I was, and am. I know how terrible the world is. But still. I want to tell the whole story not for any kind of pity, but for the hope that telling it will make me stop trying to relive it, will make my past go away. Even though I have spent my entire adulthood creating a different kind of life for myself, my head, my soul, my spirit—whatever you want to call it—is still stuck in the mire of my childhood.

Also an important detail to add here is that Mom's stalker Bates sometimes parked in our driveway, and that did actually add to the scariness of the house.

When my parents' divorce was finalized, my mom bought a town house at 125 East Ninety-Fourth Street. This sounds like a posher situation than it actually was. Eighties New York was fun and slightly scary. It was not fancy. Fancy people lived in the country, fancy people lived in Greenwich and Westport. The people who raised their kids in New York during the eighties and nineties were kind of crazy. Eighties New York was dirty, streets lined in garbage, walls covered in graffiti.

My mother bought the house with the hopes that it would be the place she started her new life. She was big on "new lives," but those lives were always tinged with drinking, and sometimes drugs. The house looked like all the other narrow brownstone houses on the sloping block, but it wasn't the same. She painted the front door bubblegum pink. People who visited the house said it looked like a haunted bordello, but that wasn't because the house was haunted—that was because my mother had terrible taste. She put floral wallpaper in each room. Later, she'd hang paintings of people having sex (bequeathed by the sexologists who would move into the basement) on that floral wallpaper.

The townhouse was broken into several times. Once they locked Mom's assistant in a room while they robbed the place, stealing some of her cheap jewelry. But in the eighties and early nineties, crime was just kind of something we learned to live with. In school, the teachers would give us little lectures about what to do and how to protect ourselves when we would (inevitably) get mugged.

Each time the house was robbed, I found myself thinking magical thoughts. Could I prevent the robberies? I became OCD. I started compulsively checking everything—checking locks, checking under the bed, checking the alarm. Could this prevent the break-ins? I had two closets in my room, and every night I would check those closets, and then I would make sure the windows were closed and the shades were drawn.

I hadn't entirely remembered that the house was haunted until a reporter friend sent me a clip he'd found in a dusty microfiche machine somewhere in the bowels of the huge limestone New York Public Library. Until then, my childhood home's hauntedness had been kind of blurred from memory, but as soon as I read the smudged newspaper print, I remembered the feelings of dread it generated. From the *New York Post*:

"The writer Erica Jong lived for five years in an East Side

brownstone that she is convinced was haunted. 'I always had splitting headaches, and I woke up at night having the wrong dreams, dreams belonging to someone else,' says Ms. Jong. She asked a psychic to visit the house and perform an exorcism. But the psychic begged off, saying the work is just too hard. Instead, the healer promised to make a psychic house call in the middle of the night to take away the bad spirits."

I posted that quote on Twitter. Afterward, a woman contacted me, writing that her parents had bought that house from my mother. Apparently, her mother had also lost her mind there. Her parents subsequently got divorced. Maybe the house was cursed, maybe we were. The house got to us all eventually.

As for dreams, I never had someone else's dreams. My own dreams were scary enough. My dreams were filled with my mother's real-life stalker, Bates, who called on the phone and had these weird conversations with me. I would hear him breathing on the phone. He'd ask me about the weather. Sometimes I would just hear the music from the radio in his pocket. Sometimes I would hear clicking on the line. (No caller ID back then.) Sometimes my nanny Margaret would run over and grab the phone out of my hand and slam it down. Sometimes she'd call the police on Bates. He'd show up at our house, that weird little radio always in his pocket.

Sometimes I'd answer the door and we'd stand there and talk. I remember thinking he wasn't that much older than I was, but that he was very strange looking. Sorry to say this, but you knew just by looking at him that he wasn't quite right. He knew my name. He knew random stuff about me. Did my mother talk to him or encourage him? Sometimes he'd go away. Then he'd come back, like herpes.

It is important to mention as frequently as possible that I came from a family of writers and I could not read. Like not at all. I was also very bad at learning. Here I was, a child and grandchild of famous writers, and I couldn't fucking read a sentence. The words swirled around, the letters made no sense. All of it seemed completely impossible to understand. I would stare at books and try to figure out what the words said. Except for my cousin, I was the only dyslexic in the family. There was always a sense that I wasn't supposed to be dyslexic because my parents were, you know, *writers*.

"I knew you were dyslexic because you just couldn't figure out your letters," my dad told me recently. After the divorce, I saw him only every other weekend. When we were together, we would do math flashcards and he would try to teach me my multiplication tables. My mother never did flashcards with me. She hired tutors, countless tutors, endless shrinks. With the shrinks I'd play with dollhouses and complain about how much I hated Cash, whom Mom called Dart in some of her books. Is Dart even really a name? (Is Cash?)

My dyslexia led to my being asked to leave Dalton in third grade. It was crushing to my father: my aunt—his sister—had gone to Dalton, and another aunt had taught at Dalton. Dalton was the height of fancy jewelry for my family. But I floundered. I just couldn't keep up. I just couldn't read as hard as I tried to read. I was put in special groups and talked about in whispers. I remember everyone else moving into normal reading groups and me staying with the learning specialist. I remember watching in wonder and awe at how people actually learned to read. I remember thinking that I could *will* myself into reading and then being truly ashamed of the fact that those letters didn't make any sense.

Eventually, in middle school, I just memorized all the words. I really just did it out of desperation and because I couldn't stand feeling stupid anymore.

I always wondered if my mom was disappointed by my dyslexia, and by the fact that I wasn't a great student like she was, but I will say that she never let me know it if she felt that way. Of course, she must have been totally devastated that I just couldn't read, that I had to go from tutor to tutor, but she was really great about not ever criticizing me for my learning disability, or for my lack of academic success.

My mom was convinced that I was a genius, like completely convinced that not being able to read or do math or figure out the months wasn't any reflection of my intelligence—if anything, all of this was proof that my brilliance was too unconventional, too unorthodox to be understood by average people in the average, stupid, boring, ordinary world. In this regard at least, I would never have been so supportive a mom.

As I was in the process of getting counseled out of Dalton, Mom needed to find a school for me to go to. Finding a second private school to attend when the first private school doesn't want you is kind of very difficult.

I went to an interview at an all-girls school called Hewitt. For some reason, during the interview, I jumped up and down and basically had a fit in front of the headmaster. Mom was really embarrassed by my behavior but was ultimately extremely nice about it. Later in the day, when my nanny picked me up at Dalton, I told her what had happened earlier at Hewitt. Margaret made me feel bad about myself. "You're too old to be so bratty," she said. But my mother never said anything like that.

When I got home my mom was forgiving about my little fit,

but I knew it pained her that I was such a fuckup, such a mess, so incapable of being the student she had been.

Needless to say, I did not get into Hewitt.

(And this was the second time I had made a huge, embarrassing public scene. That first time had happened when I was very young and had fallen off my pony (name: Heavenly Hash), and needed a tetanus shot. I would not let the pediatrician give me one. He literally had to chase me around the office while I screamed my head off. Afterward, Mom said I had to write the words "I will not make a public scene" one hundred times on a yellow legal pad—but she let me stop at fifty.)

Anyway, I think it was really hard for someone like my mom, who had been such a good student, and who cared so much about education, to have a dyslexic daughter, but she never made me feel that I was a disappointment or not smart.

So, no, the house on Ninety-Fourth wasn't haunted: it was me. I was haunted by my parents' divorce, by my mother's drinking, by the fear that she would abandon me, by my overall stupidity. The bad spirits weren't coming from the house; they were coming from inside me.

Ghosts would have at least been some company in the house. There was never anyone in the house, and it always felt empty—a house filled with empty rooms, beds no one slept in, baths no one bathed in, and a dining room no one ate in. Every day, I came home to silence. I would go upstairs to Margaret's room and sit on the floor and watch television. My TV-viewing started at 3:15 and I used to know the schedule by heart: *Facts of Life*, *The Cosby Show*, *Diff'rent Strokes*, *WKRP in Cincinnati*. *Three's Company* came on later because it was dirty. I would sometimes break for dinner and sometimes not. (Dinner was usually a TV dinner in one of those foil trays, warmed up by Margaret.) These shows taught me what normal American life was like. I was like one of those foreign kids who learned English from TV, except I wasn't learning English. I was learning how to pretend to be a normal human child with a normal childhood, with siblings, with friends, and with parents.

For most of my childhood, Mom was traveling. There wasn't an invitation to a book fair or festival, speaking engagement, or interview that she'd decline. And when Mom *was* at home in New York, she was out dancing at Nell's, or fighting with Elaine, the owner of Elaine's, the famous (infamous?) restaurant on the Upper East Side. Sometimes people would come to dinner at our house: writers, agents, and various other New York figures, but fewer than you'd think. Mom wasn't great at making new friends or figuring out how to be popular. She was so trapped in her own narcissism that she wasn't really able to fake it for a conversation. She was also even then wildly repetitive and would often launch into her speeches and forget to listen to the other person.

Because she was, at the time, famous, people gave her a lot of leeway. But such allowances are a favor to no one, least of all to the narcissist. Being able to get away with everything made her, in fact, very boring. (I am reminded of this when I watch the way people like Elon Musk exist in the world: you need someone in your life who can tell you when you're full of shit.)

Sometimes I'd be in bed and Mom would knock on my door, sometimes drunk, and sometimes just tipsy, but always smelling of the most wonderful perfume. My bedroom on Ninety-Fourth Street was arguably the best room in the house—second floor, three huge windows, high, high ceilings. She'd peek her head into my room and stage-whisper, "I have *New York Super Fudge Chunk!*" And then she'd ask me if I wanted to go into her room and watch TV with her, on her bed.

This was the best thing ever in the whole world. Margaret gave me a crazy strict bedtime, but when Mom would ask me to watch TV with her, I would run right up the stairs to her room and watch TV and eat ice cream until my stomach hurt. I loved those nights so much.

Mom would let me stay home from school the following day. She was a firm believer in mental health days. Margaret didn't believe in mental health days, but my glamorous mom didn't believe in the rules. Rules were for boring unfamous people who balanced their checkbooks. Rules were for normal people. My mother was not normal nor did she want to be.

Two infamous/notorious sexologists, Phyllis and Eberhard Kronhausen, eventually moved into our ground floor, after their landlord Shirley MacLaine kicked them out of her apartment on Central Park West. It was nice to have someone else in the house even if they were old and creepy and weirdly thin and leathery. They took handfuls of vitamins every day. Eventually, they moved back to their farm in Costa Rica. They told me I should come visit them and I never did. They left the basement filled with erotic paintings as a gift to my mom. Most of the kids I knew growing up found the house, and our art, fascinating. My friend Ruthy couldn't believe there was a painting of naked lesbians having sex at the top of the stairs. My other friend Juno wasn't as shocked as Ruthy, but that was only because her parents were psychoanalysts and she had a male nanny.

*

HOW TO LOSE YOUR MOTHER

Much of my feminist mother's time was occupied by men. But maybe, come to think of it, this shouldn't come as all that much of a surprise to readers of her fiction. After all, in *Fear of Flying*, she wrote, "Underneath it all, you longed to be annihilated by love, to be swept off your feet, to be filled up by a giant prick spouting sperm, soapsuds, silk and satin, and of course money."

And of course money.

But my mom wasn't obsessed with money. If anything, she was super self-destructive when it came to money. She was always a bit snobbish. So she might not have cared if a man was rich, but she would definitely care if he was smart.

She was always in love with someone. More often than not, it was a problematic man, a "no-account" count, a married writer who lived in Brooklyn, or a drug-addicted B-list actor. Between her divorce from my father (husband number three) and her marriage to my stepfather (husband number four) there were numerous fiancés. I couldn't help but envision each one as a possible father. It would take me years to understand that the worst possible thing you could do to a kid was introduce her to possible stepfathers on a daily basis. But my feminist mother was always looking for someone to save her, someone to get her out of her own head.

There was the wine merchant who kept his wine under the Thames. He had tax problems (but then again so did Mom) and he said he was going to build Mom an office on the property of his Connecticut house. He had an architect make up a little blueprint of the guest cottage office, but, bizarrely, it didn't have windows. Mom went around telling everyone that the wine merchant wanted to put her in a windowless house. She had asked him for the office, and he went so far as to have designs made for one, and then she mocked him for his efforts.

Wasn't that cruel?

So much of our life was like that. We'd meet someone, and then they'd become a joke. They'd become copy. To quote my mother's frenemy Nora Ephron, everything was copy. Real life didn't really exist. It was all just fodder for the next book.

These men were like a Ferris wheel of potential lives. If she picked one man, we could end up living in a dilapidated palazzo in Venice. If she picked a different man, we could end up in a modern beach house in Malibu. There was the nebbishy guy who had a daughter slightly older than I was. Maybe she'd be my sister and she'd keep me from being bullied at school. We all went on a golfing vacation to Hilton Head—the most WASPy, most boring, most Republican place on earth. Can you imagine? That great disrupter Erica Jong in *Hilton Head*? I watched TV the whole time. There was the married CEO who wanted to leave his wife for Mom. But he turned out to be a Republican, so of course he got mocked and scorned for that.

There was the magazine editor who took her out dancing in SoHo. He turned out to be gay. There was the TV host (one date). There was always some guy, and then there was always some other guy waiting in the wings. Sometimes they actually dumped *her* and she would be shocked. She did not take getting dumped well at all.

I mostly hated my mother's boyfriends, and they mostly hated me. (Generally speaking, they ignored me.) But there was one who was sincerely nice to me. He was actually interested in who I was. I think of him as the one who got away. His name was David and he would take me for ice cream. He would talk to me about school and he'd try to teach me about art. We would go for walks. David was an architect from South Carolina who seemed desperate for a family. But then we weren't much of a family, my mom and me.

Even as a little kid, I noted how strange it was to be with an adult who wasn't being paid to be with me. Most of the time the adults around me were paid to be with me. I was their job. Perhaps it was better that way, less complicated.

And where did those potential dads go? Did they end up finding other lives? Did they end up having other stepdaughters? Did they ever think about us? Even at the time I knew it was extremely strange to have all these adult men wander in and out of my life like actors auditioning for the part of playing the man who would eventually marry my mom.

Did I mention those men ended up in the books? Because they did. Everyone ended up in her novels. Even, and especially, me. She sometimes denied it, occasionally she admitted it, which is how I knew I wasn't going crazy. It was very obvious to anyone outside of her very close circle of friends. Anyone who knew her knew that everything that happened went right into the books. Names were changed to make everything a little more pretentious, but some things were almost reported verbatim, and sometimes they were combined with weird hodgepodges of fantasies she had about other people. But the one thing that always happened was that she was the hero, always and forever.

I was eleven when Mom decided to marry Ken. They'd been going out for exactly ninety days. It was not my mother's first engagement, that year. But for whatever reason they decided to get married. They got married in Vermont. It was March, the muddy season. The ceremony took place in the parking lot behind the humble ski condo Ken bought when he was living with the girlfriend who preceded Mom.

The rehearsal dinner the night before the wedding was at a restaurant in Vermont about thirty minutes from the ski condo. The dinner was jovial. Everyone (except for me) was happy. There was a lot of toasting, a lot of optimism—which was perhaps unfounded, given that this was her fourth marriage and his third. There was also, of course, quite a lot of drunkenness. Mom, as was her wont, her habit, her compulsion, gave a drunken toast, and Ken did, too. There was much merriment to go around, but I wasn't so merry, not at all.

I was worried. I was upset because I had liked the previous boyfriend, David, the architect who was looking for a daughter. But mostly I was sad because they were threatening to fire Margaret. Though I was absolutely too old for a nanny, I had never been without her. She had raised me as her own. She taught me to pray. She took me to her Catholic church. In fact, she raised me Catholic, which in hindsight was a bit weird.

I loved Margaret more than anyone. More, even, than my mother.

Right before the wedding weekend, when Mom told me Margaret needed to go, I wept.

Given that I was the only child of an alcoholic narcissist, I was allowed to behave in a very bratty way and almost always got what I wanted. Well, not *everything* I wanted, but other stuff, stuff I could *get*. I believed that I could manipulate her into letting Margaret stay. So I was baffled when it became clear that I was not going to get my way. Usually if I made a big enough fuss, I could get what I wanted, a trait that made me an unbearable child.

"Margaret *wants* to go," Mom had said. "She *wants* to retire. She needs to be with her own family now."

I was completely floored. How could she want to leave me?

HOW TO LOSE YOUR MOTHER

I want to take a minute here to remind readers that most normal people would have quit years ago. Between my dyslexia, my OCD (which was starting to get really bad), and my mom's drinking and occasional drug-taking, taking care of me wasn't an easy job. And Margaret was my mother—well, not really, but sort of. She was more of a mother than my own mother was, that was for sure.

Later I would learn Margaret didn't want to leave at all, and that Ken wanted to fire her because he found her annoying.

So, no, I wasn't in a great mood when Mom and I were driving home from the rehearsal dinner in the rain. And then, of course, we got lost. She had a car phone: it was the size of a brick and cost a zillion dollars and almost never worked. She started making calls on it. She called my godmother, Gerri, and told her we were lost. (How did she think Gerri could possibly help us?) Then she told her she didn't want to marry Ken.

I was, I will admit, delighted to hear this.

"I can't do it," my mom said into the phone. "I *can't* marry him. He's a son of a bitch."

I interjected:

"Don't marry him. Please. We can go to *Italy*! We can take a *trip*!"

She glanced over at me. "Oh, I'm not going to marry him, Molly, don't worry," she said. And then into the gigantic phone she said, "I *hate* him."

Somehow, despite the drizzle and the dark, we made it back to the ski condo. Mom and Ken screamed at each other all night long. The next day, they got married. Then they went on a very long honeymoon. They lied and said they would try to convince Margaret to stay.

My mother and I moved into Ken's apartment. Mom sold

the townhouse and told *New York* magazine that she didn't think the ghosts there would be interested in the new owners.

Ken's apartment was in one of those white brick buildings built in the late fifties, during the brief period when white brick was fashionable. The building had doormen who wore gloves, and there was a driveway. It was fancy in a tacky way my mom would have hated earlier in her life. Bohemian people didn't live in buildings like that, but Mom wasn't bohemian anymore. She was a shape-shifter, a woman who lived the life of the man she was currently with. Ken loved this building, and didn't want to leave, so we moved in, on the twenty-seventh floor. My room had windows that opened wide enough to jump out of.

Ken loved Mom, like *loved*. The rest of the world barely existed, mostly their reality was just their love for each other. I could tell I wasn't really going to be a part of this new life. (Do I sound bitter?) I could sense that Ken wasn't going to be much of a father to me. I recognized in him a kindred spirit, though not in a good way. He was loud. He was blustery. He was used to getting his own way. He thought he was always right. He ate Steak-umms for breakfast in his bathrobe.

All these years later, I thank God for Ken. Had he not come along I would have never survived my childhood, I would have been eclipsed by my mother's need for me. She had that thing famous people have where they can't be alone. Also, despite the fact that most writers (a terribly sad bunch of individuals) feel alive only when they are alone and working, she was terrified of the empty room. More Erica Jong paradoxes to add to the pile. Ken actually came along at the exactly right time. A minute later, I would have drowned in her old opaque neediness.

They bought another apartment in the building. I didn't

want to move into the apartment because my beloved Margaret would have to sleep in a small room off the kitchen: *the maid's room*. Yes, they continued lying to me about keeping Margaret. This new maid's-room situation seemed very mean—she would feel unvalued, unappreciated, unloved—though it was not as mean as their true plan. I begged Mom and Ken not to buy the apartment. But of course they did, and right after we moved in, they finally fired Margaret. I was bereft. I wept. I had lost my best, and only, friend.

I know how fucked up that is.

My mother put up pink-and-white-striped wallpaper in my new room. The previous owners had used the room as their study, and it had these enormous shutters that my mother painted white. Nothing ever looked right in my new room because my mom had terrible taste.

But at least I had my own telephone line, which was the height of privilege for an eighties kid. The phone was neon. I had—ultimate power—a phone line I could use whenever I wanted. I didn't have to share a phone with anyone else.

The apartment had been owned by the Chunky candy people. The Chunky candy bar was in my estimation the worst candy bar—a weird big square, but not as big as a 3 Musketeers and not as yummy as a Snickers. No caramel. No crunch. Just chocolate, nuts, and, bafflingly, raisins. It came in a silver wrapper. I remember meeting the Chunky people when Mom and Ken bought the place. The guy was jovial and jolly, funny and weird. He seemed to know that Mom was a celebrity of some sort. When we came to see the apartment before we bought it, they didn't offer us any candy. I didn't understand how the people who made their fortune in candy didn't have any candy for us. For years afterward, my parents would call him the Chunky Candy Bar Guy. I think they moved to Florida. This seems completely right for a thousand different reasons.

Imagine making your fortune on the world's worst candy bar.

The idea of buying the apartment from a candy man was, in my mind, pretty ironic. Although I don't think Mom and Ken appreciated the significance, I was sort of struck by it. I never got over being a fat kid (neither did my father), and never got over the idea that a fat kid moved into an apartment that candy built.

4

The weird thing about the shit hitting the fan is that it's oddly liberating. So much of American life is faking it, pretending everything is all right, pretending your postpartum depression is just something everyone goes through . . . but there's something freeing about a bomb going off in the middle of your life, about your worst fears coming true. There is something amazing about knowing the worst-case scenario is finally upon you. It's oddly liberating.

Matt and I were lying in bed the night before the surgery. We were having one of those pre-cancer-surgery conversations. I was also trying to go to sleep.

"You know Sloan Kettering is where all my aunts and uncles died," Matt offered.

Was he being funny? His sense of humor is wildly tuned and deft—and grim—but I wasn't sure if he was being darkly humorous, or if he was truly worried that he was going to die. I was too afraid to ask.

We arrived at the hospital at 8:15 the following morning.

After many delays, Matt went in for surgery at 2:45 p.m. I left the hospital. I walked home, to get some air and to clear my head. Sometimes the magnitude of what was happening was lost on me. Sometimes it was decidedly not. My walk home was sunny, but cold. Once at home, I took a bath. The hospital called. It was now Hour Two. From a nurse, I received what could turn out to be the first of many pieces of bad news: they couldn't do the surgery laparoscopically. This could mean nothing, but it could also theoretically mean that Matt was going to die.

Twenty minutes later, the surgeon called me. It was one of those conversations that probably lasted only a few minutes, but it felt like hours. There was something ominous in his voice and I tried to get as much information as possible from him, but it was a struggle. I can always detect *that thing* in someone's voice; I can always tell when someone wants to say more but can't. (Maybe everyone has this knack, or maybe I'm some kind of brilliant genius at dealing with people.) This doctor is a man who is accustomed to delivering bad news, and he's skilled at modulating his tone. He reiterated that they weren't able to do the surgery laparoscopically. Thank you, but I knew this, because the nurse had already told me. But wait, there was more.

"We think it's the bad cancer," he said.

I knew that as long as I live, I would never forget this moment. Where I was standing in my apartment, what I was wearing. I will relive this moment over and over again, for eternity.

"O*kay*," I said.

"And we want to remove his gallbladder," the doctor added.

What? I don't even know what a gallbladder *is*. Where is it? What does it do?

"Does his gallbladder have cancer?" I asked.

"We don't *think* so," he said. "But it's inflamed and hard."

I looked out the window. Across the street is a very fancy apartment building they've been working on for years. Someday very, very rich people will move into this building, into those apartments. People for whom ten million dollars is a rounding error. Or, more accurately, they may never move into these apartments. They may use these apartments as a means to get money out of China or Russia or some other country. Many of these very rich people may be criminals of one sort or another. And the apartments these rich criminals will buy will make our apartment more valuable. I was thinking that this—all of this, all of it—might not end well. This might indeed end badly. Like really badly.

"When you got in there," I asked the doctor. I was trying to hedge. I was trying to ask questions in a way that didn't make me sound like an asshole. "When you got in there, did you see cancer everywhere?"

"No," he said. We had been warned that they might find huge lumps of cancer everywhere. That had not happened. "But I need your permission to remove the gallbladder."

I gave the surgeon permission to remove my husband's gallbladder, an organ I don't think I've ever spent more than a second thinking about. It's a joke organ, right? The gallbladder: butt of all jokes. Matt's anesthetized body was now gaping open on the operating table. I was thinking about how incurably disgusting—yet how miraculous—the human body is. And I was thinking about my husband's weird, hard gallbladder.

My AA sponsor, Susan C., called me. She was one of the few people in the world who knew what was going on with Matt. She has known me since I was a teenager and I rely on her wisdom, insight, and sanity. She told me that it was okay to be angry. She said that I'm allowed to say, "This *sucks*."

I realized that I was an object of pity in Susan's eyes, and I also realized that I didn't even hate being an object of pity.

"The fact that you have to live both the apex of your career and the low plex of this is something," Susan said.

Was this the apex of my career? God, I hoped not. And was this the low plex? Not necessarily. Things could get both better and worse.

"I've been so lucky my whole life," I said. "It's okay."

"I don't really think you've been all that lucky," Susan said.

The calculus had changed once again from lucky wife to future widow. How was I going to tell Matt if he had the bad cancer?

We hadn't told my mother or my stepfather about the cancer stuff. They seemed unable to process it. Would it be okay to never tell them? That seemed fucked up, but it also sort of made a lot of sense. My left temple had been hurting. Was I dying, too?

The surgeon called back to say that maybe it *was* the good cancer after all. We wouldn't have a definitive answer for another week, but at least I was no longer a forty-four-year-old widow. Not tonight, at least. Now I could imagine growing old with my husband. Growing old now seems not a horrible burden, but a great gift.

I looked at Instagram. Why not? No bad news there, right? Only photoshopped and airbrushed bullshit: roses, rainbows, and sunshine. But my friend Mandy Stein posted a picture of her sister, Samantha. Today, February 1, would have been Sam's fiftieth birthday. She died of a brain tumor a decade ago.

Mandy and Sam's father is (was? he's dead now too) the music mogul Seymour Stein. He founded Sire Records and discovered Madonna and the Talking Heads. Sam was maybe five feet tall. She was a few years older than I was and was one of those people who was always kind of a mess, but who also had this fabulous glamorous life. Until, that is, she was about thirty-eight, and was diagnosed with an inoperable brain tumor. The horrible irony of Sam's birthday being the same day as Matt's surgery was not lost on me.

Mandy and Sam's mother had died a few years before Sam got sick: murdered by her assistant with a weighted yoga stick in her Fifth Avenue apartment. These people had all the money and power in the world, and they were surrounded by excess upon excess, and fame, and it turned out they still died tragically, and none of it could save them.

The thing that made me so obsessed with my mother wasn't her fame or lack of it. The thing that made us so close was that I was her only child. Other only children know what it means to be your parents' only link to immortality. You are the end of the line. There is no one else but you, you are their only shot at forever. If you disappear, they disappear, too. You are the last link, the last little bit of flesh and bone that can carry on the family genes, name, freckles, DNA, and genetic diseases. If an only child dies without having children, the genetic line is dead. Perhaps it was better that way, with my line of alcoholism and depression and Tay-Sachs and Canavan disease. Maybe it was time for my little gene puddle to evaporate.

But when I was twenty-four, I got pregnant by accident.

When my mother got pregnant with me at thirty-six (not by accident), the first thing her editor at New American Library did was to take out a life insurance policy on her; not exactly a vote of confidence.

When I got pregnant by accident, the first thing I did was

write an essay about it for *The New York Times*, an essay that feels really dated now, but here's a not completely embarrassing paragraph from it:

> I used to think I would have my first child at 41. I used to think I would be the one making those surreptitious trips to Paris. But the truth was that I just didn't know myself at all. I hate Paris. I hate flying. Maybe having a baby will slow my career; maybe I will have to spend more time than I want at a Y.M.C.A. pool and less at the rooftop pool of Soho House. But, wait. I've never been there anyway.

And so I didn't have an abortion at twenty-four. I had a child. I had a son. I was now the mother of an only child. He was our little genius. We stared at him. We worshipped him. He was the only child, the only grandson. When we wanted more children, we learned that we carried two Jewish genetic diseases each, Matt and I. We puzzled over what to do. Any child we would have was doomed to a twenty-five percent chance of suffering from Canavan disease—a degenerative disorder like ALS—and likely not living past five or six. The idea of signing up for a death sentence, or a second-trimester abortion, seemed insane to me. For a while we were at a stalemate. Maybe we shouldn't have more children. Maybe we didn't need any more kids, maybe our lives were perfect already. After all, the planet was clearly dying. Wasn't bringing a child into this mess kind of selfish?

In the end, the need to continue on won out.

Our twin embryos were sliced and diced and grown in dishes and ultimately hatched in a lab in New Jersey and implanted in me. A girl and a boy. We were thrilled. I remember the phone call as if it were yesterday. "Baby A is a boy and Baby B is a girl."

All I wanted was a girl.

And then various things happened to me that happen to women pregnant with twins, the worst of which was gestational diabetes, but I also had rashes of indeterminate origin and intermittent vomiting.

And then one day I went into the hospital for a planned C-section. It was supposed to be normal. Everything was supposed to be normal.

It was one of those perfect blue January days, no clouds and the air was cold. I walked down Fifth Avenue to the hospital for my procedure. I remember being sure everything would go exactly as planned, because people don't die in childbirth anymore. Before I went into surgery, I said to Matt, "The twins may end up in the NICU because they are twins and sometimes things like that happen with twins, but don't worry. I'll be fine. Make sure you go see them."

The surgery started as planned surgeries at teaching hospitals often do. Multiple doctors were milling about, making jokes. They told the students where they would cut through the skin. They drew lines on my flesh with markers. Doctors mused about where they would eventually stitch up my "teaching" body. There was talk about my first C-section scar, from my first child's birth. "Did you *see* the scar tissue here?" one of the doctors asked one of the students. It was then that it occurred to me they were cutting into me.

"You're going to feel a little bit of tugging," the doctor declared. I wondered if the tugging was the cutting through of my flesh. I thought about the doctors getting together and deciding to use the word "tugging" instead of something else. "Tugging" sounds a lot less scary than "slicing through you like cold cuts," right?

There was tugging, and then there was panic, and maybe some other things in between, but I don't remember. I don't remember the moment we went from casual "teaching" to keeping the mother from bleeding out on the table. One of the nurses screamed at all the young doctors to leave. I think one of my doctors shouted, "Everybody out!" It was at that moment when it occurred to me that I could conceivably die.

As someone who suffers from anxiety, I spend much of my life obsessed with the possibility of the worst-case scenario. Now I was *living* the worst-case scenario.

One of the doctors said with just a little too much edge, "We might have to put her under," and that the nurses should start putting the IVs in my neck (although it turned out that what she meant was sort of more the collarbone area). One of the other doctors mused, also with an anxious tone that did not fill me with confidence, that I was going to need some of my universal-recipient AB-positive blood for a transfusion because I was losing so much blood.

The daughter I had always wanted, her placenta was growing into my uterine wall. The doctors told me they couldn't stop the bleeding.

One of my doctors—the serious, thin one—shouted, "Someone get a mop." She couldn't get sure footing while she was stitching. I looked over at my husband, who was wearing a surgical mask. This was before the once-in-a-century pandemic, and people didn't wear surgical masks like they do now. I could see the fear and terror in his eyes. I knew that he was not prone to panic and this was not what I wanted to see. I was twenty-nine. I grew up a druggie and an alcoholic. I always thought I would die tragically, but not in a hospital. I thought it would happen in a cheap hotel on the Strip after snorting something I was sure was cocaine but turned out to be heroin. That's how someone like me dies.

I didn't die. I didn't even see any tunnel or bright white light. They stopped the bleeding, they sewed up things as best they could. They saved my uterus, but the doctor also casually mentioned that I couldn't have any more children. Later, I would ask one of the doctors—the thin, serious one—why they didn't do a hysterectomy. "Sometimes you just have to close the patient up" was the no-nonsense reply. So I would have no more children, but I did have my uterus, a misshaped fragile organ that was now purely decorative. Me and my purely decorative uterus would live another day.

A friend of my in-laws picked me up at the hospital. He regarded me gravely, as if he were considering a ghost. I was painfully, deeply white from the lack of blood. I remember how much it hurt to sit in the seat in the car. I remember everything about my pain. But I don't remember where my mom was. Maybe she was there in the car, too?

Back at home, I just couldn't believe how profoundly tired I was. The doctors told me I had lost so much blood it would take me a while to get back to normal.

I had bruises on both sides of my neck where they had inserted IVs. Everything hurt like hell. The bruises on my neck were more pronounced because my skin was ghostly white. For the first few weeks, my husband and I were terrified of the twins.

They had almost killed me, after all. Of course, it wasn't them, they were little blameless babies, but it often felt hard to tell.

Sometimes I would touch the bruises on my neck just to feel the weird dull pain of a healing bruise.

Matt and I were both completely traumatized. I had almost died and had somehow managed not to. We'd just sit there staring at each other. Sometimes he would just look at me and touch me to make sure I was still there, and not some kind of widower's hallucination. My eldest son was no longer our only link to the future. Now there were three. And now I had a girl.

I used to think I would never ever have a daughter. My mother used to tease me that I would have three boys. I always desperately wanted a daughter. I suppose I wanted to fix all the things I'd done wrong, or all the things my mother had done wrong.

Later, my mother would write about my birth experience in her novel *Fear of Dying*. In this story, I am a peripheral character, the daughter of the heroine of the novel, Isadora Wing, my mother's alter ego. Just as in real life. The peripheral character. The daughter. In this book my name is Glinda (a reminder that my mother had wanted to name me Belinda):

"As for Glinda, she delighted in telling and retelling the story of her giving birth—embellishing with each retelling. Her labor got longer and longer, her bleeding more and more excessive, her heroism greater."

I wouldn't have seen the paragraph if my husband hadn't read the book. I don't read my mother's books. I need to protect myself. But the fact was that I almost died and my mom thought it either didn't happen, or that it did happen but that I was exaggerating and trying to make myself a hero. Imagine that. Imagine that the worst thing that's ever happened to you is portrayed as a figment of your own imagination. *By your own mother.*

I never thought of not bleeding to death as an act of heroism. I wasn't a hero for not dying in childbirth, I was just, as so many times in my life, lucky. But that's the problem with being lucky, with being born into a lucky situation—you know that the luck, like fame, is only temporary. Luck runs out for everyone sooner or later.

5

It was now Wednesday, a week after the surgery, and Matt was home with a drain and a bad attitude. We were still waiting for the pathology report. The pathology would dictate the next few days, weeks, years. The pathology would dictate the rest of our calculations. What if Matt stopped making money? (He had continued working this whole time.) And then there was the anxiety which for some reason had become enormous in my head: Would Matt outlive his powerful father, the one who has largely dominated his life—the father who lived through both the Holocaust *and* Great Depression? The thing about Matt's dad was that he was *perfect*. Stu was wildly successful. He was a genius. He had read everything. He could talk about anything and he had grown some of the most interesting companies in the world. He was also a serious environmentalist and was deeply kind. I needed Stu to live forever. But I also needed Matt to outlive him.

Pathology finally came back. We awaited the results during Matt's postsurgical visit. We were sitting in the exam room. This part of Sloan Kettering is in an office building in Midtown, next to the so-called Lipstick Building, where Bernie Madoff's offices were. The doctor entered the room. He told us that Matt has the "neuroendocrine kind" of cancer. It sounded bad, but this was actually what we wanted to hear because it's the "good" pancreatic cancer. (Although it's also the one that killed Steve Jobs.) We should have been delighted. This meant that death wasn't imminent for Matt.

Then the surgeon had something to add.

"It's spread to the lymph nodes."

We paused.

"It *is* cancer," the surgeon added.

We've had a very hard time saying the word "cancer" since the diagnosis. We've tried to use other words because we're good with words.

We didn't really know what to say. Since I am an idiot, I said something idiotic. "But this is *good* news, right?" I asked. "This is the 'good cancer.'"

Matt gave me a dirty look. Later, I would learn that Matt really hated it when I called it the "good cancer."

The surgeon seemed chipper enough. He said that they had a lot of different ways to treat this cancer, but because it was in the lymph nodes, there was a forty or fifty percent chance of recurrence. We deal in percentages now. The percentage of likelihood that he'll be at our oldest son's college graduation. The percentage of likelihood that he'll be at our twins' high school graduation. We have become an enormous math problem—an unsolvable math problem, in fact.

I was still pretty sure that I was going to become a widow. When you're a kid and your parents leave you, you're certain that other people will leave you, too. That's why I married Matt—dependable, very smart, very safe Matt. I knew Matt was too practical, too serious to ever leave me. I never factored in cancer. I guess I should have, though—his father's sister and brother died of cancer, and his mother's two sisters did too, and both, as I've mentioned, in their fifties. Also his cousin. Why had I assumed that the cancer would never come to him?

I got sober at nineteen because I knew that no one was there to rescue me. I got married at twenty-five because no one had ever taken care of me. Now it was my turn to take care of Matt. But how much caretaking was I even capable of?

I never thought of myself as the star of my own life, or my own childhood. From a young age, I knew my mom was writing about me. I knew it because people would come up to me and ask me very personal questions, which meant they knew things they couldn't possibly know unless someone was telling them things about me. I never knew quite what the other person knew about me. In some ways, it made me very good at talking to people; in other ways, it made me a psychopath. I never had privacy, so I never valued privacy. I just assumed everyone knew everything about me and about everyone else.

As my kids grew up, I walked the dangerous line of becoming my mother. I was careful but I still did it sometimes.

At a party, my friend Adrienne and I were talking about our children. She pointed out that I rarely wrote about my kids. A minute before, a fancy corporate lawyer in a suit had told me I had "Trump Derangement Syndrome." We hadn't even spoken yet. All I'd done was tell him my name, and "Oh, you're the one with Trump Derangement Syndrome" was the response. I stared at him. For hours afterward, I ruminated over the things I could have said, the ways I could have gotten back at him, but in the moment, all I could manage to do was laugh. I laughed because I was in my mid-forties and I was not standing up for myself. A woman in her thirties would have replied with something cutting, but I was, unfortunately, part of that odd generation for whom sexual harassment was something you just sat back and agreed with. Maybe you were wearing a skirt that showed too much skin. Maybe it *was* all your fault.

As someone with a deranged mother and stepfather, I spent a lot of time thinking about being deranged and what that meant exactly.

Anyway, Adrienne was right that I never write about my children. I'd always known that I had to protect them from myself, from this pathetical desire to show the world absolutely everything.

I was deranged. I am deranged. I am bits and pieces of a normal person and I don't want that for them. No one wants that for their kids. No amount of fame is worth turning my children into the weird hollow doll I am.

This is why I'm careful when I write about my kids, and I am the most careful when I write about my daughter. I have two sons, but I'm more protective of my daughter. I know the damage a same-sex parent can inflict, often by accident. I think about it a lot, obviously. My mom loved me so much, but she could hurt me in a way my father could not. My father was damaged by his father in a way my aunt was not.

When I was a kid, my mother published a children's picture book about me because of course she did. She told me she wrote *Megan's Book of Divorce* to help me deal with her divorce from my father. It's a crazy piece of work. A blog called *Awful Library Books* had some fun with it, referencing, among other transgressions, something called "the bizarre underwear scene." In the scene in question, I (or "Megan") am not wearing underwear. I'm kneeling before my toy box and appear to be fellating a stuffed dog (naturally, I'm looking for my missing underwear). I am given the line "I think divorce is dumb because I never remember where I left my underpants." The publishers liked the butt drawing so much they also put it on the back cover. This is not the only problem with the book.

There is the reflexive racism (one of Megan's nannies, Bessie-Lou, has "healin' hands" and takes young Megan "to meet her pastor in Harlem. Hallelujah!"). There is the fact that Megan wants her mother to kill her stepmother. There are continuity issues, there is the ever-present Erica Jong problem of unexamined privilege, but the most obvious and tragic problem: the author of the book seems to have about as much familiarity with children as she would with extraterrestrials from Mars.

Believe it or not, my mom sold the film rights to this picture book to ABC. A pilot was shot. Loretta Swit—she portrayed the character "Hot Lips" Houlihan on *M*A*S*H*—played my mother, and Keri Houlihan played me. (In one of those exceptionally weird, yet certainly meaningless, twists of fate, the fictional "Hot Lips" and the very real Keri had the same last name.) They changed the title to *Sam* because my dad threatened to sue my mom unless my name were changed. (Although my name in the book had *already* been changed to Megan. By that point in my life, I had learned not to ask too many questions.)

As another data point from the *Megan's Book of Divorce* debacle, I would like to submit this correction from a piece about me written in *The New York Times* in 2022, which, for those keeping track at home, is thirty-seven years after said sitcom. The correction was sent in by my father:

"An earlier version of this article incorrectly stated that

HOW TO LOSE YOUR MOTHER

Molly Jong-Fast's father, Jonathan Fast, sued her mother, Erica Jong, over Ms. Jong's depiction of a fictional character based on Ms. Jong-Fast and her experience with her parents' divorce. Mr. Fast's lawyer was involved in the dispute, but he did not file a lawsuit."

Have I mentioned yet that my father wanted my name changed when I was a child? He was worried that I would be kidnapped ... or at least that was the reason I heard. Getting kidnapped was more of a thing in the eighties. My friend Marci Klein (Calvin's kid—sorry to name-drop—and now a celebrated TV producer) got kidnapped by her childhood nanny in 1978 when she was ten. My father's friend's kid was kidnapped on her way to school in the eighties. I never worried too much about getting kidnapped, however. My parents weren't famous enough for me to be a kidnapping target, for starters. (Though on the upside, if I did get kidnapped, my mother's next novel would just write itself.)

When the pilot was filmed in 1985, my mother took me out of school and moved us to L.A. for a month. We lived at the Beverly Hills Hotel. I don't remember much about living in L.A. except that it was yet another time when my mom was convinced that she had made it and wouldn't have to worry about money anymore. But the show was not picked up and we went home.

We hadn't made it. My mom would still live (well), but from book to book. Mom was always convinced that someday she would make so much money that she wouldn't have to worry about money, but she was always worried about money. The more money she made the more worried she was that she wouldn't make money the next time. Sometimes she would find herself in a pickle—like the time she found out she owed a million dollars to the IRS and had to ask her dad for a loan.

After we left L.A., I started seeing one of those serious therapists with the dollhouses who made me talk about my feelings. My mother may have sent me because of the not-sleeping, or the sleepwalking (when I did sleep), or perhaps it was the OCD stuff. At any rate, there is nothing that can make a person hate their feelings more than someone earnestly demanding they talk about these feelings with you. And, boy, I hated therapy. I didn't want to talk about myself. I kept thinking about what the shrink's life was like. Did the shrink have kids? Did the shrink love her kids? Did they have dinner together? Was she a good cook? I always assumed everyone had these wonderful childhoods filled with togetherness and home-cooked meals and tennis lessons. I wished I could go live with the shrink's family.

This was around the time when I started eating. A lot. I found myself starting to identify with Augustus Gloop, the kid in *Charlie and the Chocolate Factory* who gets stuck in the chocolate-filled pipe and serves as a cautionary tale about the best of all sins, gluttony. When not gluttoning, I was talking. (I still am.)

My grandfather Howard was a famous fatphobe, and as a result my father and aunt are emaciated. When I was growing up, my dad would always tell me all the terrible things my grandfather used to call him. "Johnny Fat Fellow Fast" was his father's favorite insult. Once I saw a picture of my father on a pony wearing a funny hat. It was one of those small black-and-white photos from the 1950s. My father didn't look particularly fat, just miserable. But I've never seen one of those 1950s kid photos where the kid doesn't look particularly miserable. Dad assures me he was in fact miserable. He and I both have a certain fragility to us, a feeling that maybe the world is too much for us. I don't know if having a crushingly powerful and impressive same-sex parent made us this way or not. My father and I are in many ways the same, both children of narcissists. Children who are, essentially, afterthoughts. Sometimes we bond about this. Sometimes not.

I was fat because I ate. I ate because I didn't have anything else to do besides therapy and tutoring. Food was the only place I was happy. I loved frosting and birthday cake. I still love birthday cake. Even now, I keep thinking that there's gotta be a piece of birthday cake that will scratch that "happy childhood" itch. Fondant is still my thing.

When we got home from California, my mother went back to Europe with her boyfriend Cash. They drove down the Dalmatian coast. I stayed in New York with Margaret. On the weekends, she took me to visit with her extended family in a modest factory town in Connecticut—Danbury. Margaret and I said the Lord's Prayer every night before bed. I would kiss the Rosary before I went to bed. Sometimes I would even remember that I was Jewish.

***

They found fluid on Matt's CAT scan. This was bad. He was put back in the hospital. He was panicked. He had a high whiteblood-cell count. He had a fever. Matt was scared, and when Matt is scared, it comes out as angry.

The next day he went back into surgery. I went up to surgery with him. The interventional radiologist, a doctor wearing a mask that made him look like a duck, said that Matt would be given new drains.

I held Matt's hand.

"Are you scared?" I asked.

"I'm just sick of this," he said.

He went in and I left to do an interview with Douglas Brinkley on CNN. Doug and I talked about the environmental catastrophe in East Palestine, Ohio, where thirty-eight cars of a Norfolk Southern freight train carrying hazardous material derailed. Doug happened to do a TV interview with Mom years ago. Sometimes I go on CNN late at night—I usually arrive around 9:00—and I appear for a few segments. CNN is in Hudson Yards, an area of the city that has recently been lavishly redeveloped into all steel and marble. The area is very beautiful but seems to be a place where no one actually lives, and where people visit only when they are forced to. I was there for CNN, and then went home in the car they provided. It took more time to get the makeup off than it did to do my interview.

They drained the fluid and put Matt in a shared room on the fourteenth floor. The patient through the curtain had the bad pancreatic cancer, the normal one. It had metastasized. He was dying. He was older than Matt, but Matt was convinced they were the same age and refused to believe this. My experience at Sloan Kettering had shown me that there is no rhyme or reason to any of it. Young people sometimes have cancers that grow fast, and older people hang on. Things make no sense. It's a science but it's also not. I saw Dr. O'Reilly in the elevator, typing on her phone. She was surrounded by other doctors who followed her from patient to patient.

I got off the elevator, then got on another one: the wrong elevator. The Shabbat elevator, which stops on every floor. This seemed like as good a metaphor as any for where my life was right now: on the wrong elevator.

For a while, I wasn't telling anyone that Matt was sick and

that my parents have dementia . . . but then I decided to be honest. In truth, I could use the pity. It's also good to use as an excuse. I told total strangers. I did it because as it goes on, I feel as if I'm barely holding it together. Sometimes I feel strong, but a lot of time, just waiting in line at the grocery store will drive me over the edge. I am like the high-wire act, just trying not to fall.

It is now late winter. Mom is dirty. She won't bathe. She lives in a strange world that is both real and unreal. She has slid from the space-time continuum, her brain like a mini-science-fiction novel. The apartment smells like dog pee. Ken is wearing a diaper. He drools. Sometimes he thinks he's in France. He's covered in bruises and has been taking his medication wrong. He didn't start to be completely demented until recently. A month ago? A few months? A few weeks? It's hard to tell when he started to slip into the odd poetic otherworldliness of dementia. For a while, I could see a flicker, he was still in there but just a little.

He'd say, "I'm going upstairs for a nap."

"No, Ken, there's no upstairs here," I would say.

He'd pause. "Oh right. But there *was* an upstairs in the house I grew up in in Great Neck."

"You aren't in Great Neck, Ken," I would say.

But at some point, he entirely forgot he wasn't in Great Neck. His assistant called me to tell me he'd left her a message saying they'd just landed in L.A. He was still in the apartment.

How, and why, did I believe they could continue living this way? I don't know what I was thinking. Ken had Parkinson's, but he didn't really believe he had Parkinson's, and Mom had dementia, and she didn't really believe she had dementia . . . *or* that Ken had Parkinson's. So they both lived ignoring their diseases. He kept falling down, and she kept drinking, and no one went to the doctor, or had showers. There were the assistants, who didn't do much, and aides, who also didn't do much, and didn't know how to wash them (or how to convince them to wash). I was afraid they'd accidentally set the place on fire. I was afraid that I'd walk into their apartment one afternoon and find them both dead. But just as I did with my mom's drinking, I respected their delusions. I was a professional delusion-respecter.

At dinner one night I got a call from one of the assistants my mother and stepfather have kept because they're both planning to go back to work. But the truth is they will never go back to work. I can't tell them this because they don't listen to me. Even now they don't listen to me. They've always found me boring and hopelessly square. They think that because I got sober at nineteen I don't understand anything.

"The aides want to take Ken to the hospital," the assistant said.

He had just been in the hospital last week. But he got home and kept falling. Ken kept thinking he could walk, and move properly, but then he would fall out of bed. He was in the stage of Parkinson's where the dementia has convinced him that his body can do things that it absolutely cannot do, like get out of bed.

I am not ready for the Old People in the Emergency Room stage of life, particularly since I just spent the previous week at Sloan Kettering with my husband while he had thirty percent of his pancreas and spleen removed, not to mention a hundred percent of his gallbladder. The doctor said there was a twenty percent chance that the spleen would leak. And then it did. There's that math again, the math none of us seem able to outrun.

The aide told me that Ken was being taken back to New York Hospital. While Sloan Kettering is wonderful and filled with clean everything and women who want you to not cry and tell you cheerful things, New York Hospital is dirty. Next to Ken was a guy who was handcuffed to his bed. A cop sat in the chair next to him. To be honest, the guy in the handcuffs looked like someone I knew from my AA meetings. The tattoos looked familiar. Was he Russ from AA? I really wanted to wake him up and ask him, but that's not the kind of thing you can be wrong about.

I left Ken with his aide. Of course we were paying for an aide. We were paying for everything all the time.

I had to go check in on my mother.

When I arrived at her apartment, she was wearing a half-open hot-pink bathrobe. I wish I could report this was a new thing, but every man I've ever dated has seen my mother naked. She's always wearing a half-open bathrobe.

"Where's Ken?" she asked.

"He's at the hospital, Mom. You know that."

"Should I go there and check on him?"

"*No*, Mom," I said. "Absolutely not."

She gave me a funny look.

"You know, Ken and I are so close," she said. "He's never liked me to be with other people. He was always so jealous." This was true, oh was it ever. "He never wanted to share me with anyone. It was just us."

"I *know*," I said.

I did in fact very much know.

"But it was okay," my mom continued, "because I always had my writing. He always kept me from you, though."

Ken came home in an ambulette. The aide who had been with him at the hospital returned with him. I met them down in the lobby. I didn't want to go upstairs again. I just went home.

And then there was Matt. He still had the drain. His pancreas was still leaking fluid.

***

Maybe I was thinking we could go on like that, with both of them in denial of their diseases, with him half in this world, and half in the other magical demented plane with my mother. But one day, Ken stopped coming back to my world. One day, it became clear he was gone. That was when I understood I had to send them somewhere. But where?

I started the horrendous process of looking for a nursing home. I found one that looked okay. It was called "assisted living," but a nursing home was what it was. It was on the Upper East Side. It was also insanely expensive. So expensive that I will now take to calling it the World's Most Expensive Nursing Home. It's a place that they could afford, but just barely; however, if my mother lives to be a hundred, we'll be out of luck. I feel badly fretting about the money when I should just want her to live as long as possible, right? It's another horrible unsolvable math problem. If Erica Jong drinks a bottle of wine a day for sixty years, can she live another twenty? And what will her daughter do when she outlives the money?

But then what would her quality of life as a hundred-year-old even be? But what is the quality of any of our lives? What about our fourteen-year-old dog who is basically kept together with glue and paper clips? What is *his* quality of life? Yet another unsolvable math problem. I was told there wouldn't be math. I got a D in math in high school. I just didn't understand it. My brain didn't work that way, still doesn't.

The accountant, Art, was speaking over Zoom. Art has been my accountant my whole life. He has red hair, the color I dye mine now. I had scheduled an appointment with him to discuss how we were going to afford the World's Most Expensive Nursing Home. Maybe I could sell her jewelry?

"No," Art said. "You can't do that. You can wear it, though."

He explained that I couldn't sell her jewelry—or her art—because the sale would be taxed at a capital-gains rate. But he did have some helpful advice: wear the jewelry and hang the art in my apartment. I didn't tell Art that if I started wearing her jewelry, then I would be pretending to be her, and then, finally, once and for all, I will have assumed her identity. The one thing I have feared above and beyond all others will finally have happened.

Art, thank God, didn't know about the shit that went down in my brain. He would get very scared if he did. I have to protect other people from my brain. Maybe I've been pretending to be her this whole time? Maybe that's why I'm a writer now? Maybe that's why I still live a few blocks away from her? Maybe my whole life I've always wanted to *be* my overwhelmingly powerful mother? The fear is not that I would suffer from impostor *syndrome*—I would just be an actual imposter, full stop.

I can't do anything about my mother's drinking. I've seen my mother drunk many times. In fact, she is drunk every day. After five o'clock at home, or after lunch in Europe, she'd be drunk, although maybe not the way I used to get drunk. She wouldn't get wasted, she wouldn't vomit on the beach, or on her date (one of my most famous moves). She wasn't like me. I was a drugstore cowboy, but she was a member of polite society. I would be watching *Baywatch* with the drug dealer's girlfriend, or having nosebleeds, or wandering around the East Village, looking for an after-hours club where I could do cocaine and drink cheap beer until the sun rose. My mother was more refined. She would just fade off into the light haze of early buzzed drinking.

This is not to say that she could be counted on to be a charming drunk. Sometimes she'd get angry and start screaming. (I only saw this a few times, but it was destabilizing.) I wasn't a drunk like that, or at least I don't *think* I was. I would often just go into a blackout and then come out of it, wandering around a different city, or state, but sometimes I'd just wake up at home watching *Melrose Place*. There was no rhyme or reason to it. But I loved drinking, I loved disappearing into substances from pot to cocaine to alcohol. I loved getting out of myself.

Being the daughter, and granddaughter, of alcoholics, and as an alcoholic myself, I know all the states of drunkenness and drinking. I know the difference between two glasses of white wine consumed in rapid succession and five martinis. I know the difference between really violently drunk and slightly out-of-it spacey drunk. I know what these conditions look like from the outside and I know, I really know, how they feel from the inside.

I turned nineteen in August 1997. Two months later, in October, I was in the backseat of a Town Car with my mother. She was spraying herself with perfume. We were on the way to one of her readings.

"I need to go to rehab," I said.

On one of my last nights drinking, I walked from my apartment in the East Village to my grandparents' apartment on the Upper West Side. I was wearing platform shoes. I'd been doing cocaine and drinking Coronas for hours and hours. I walked more than five miles and finally found myself on Central Park West, outside my grandparents' building. But I realized I was just too fucked up to go inside. It was a weird moment, being too fucked up to visit my alcoholic grandma.

There in the hired car, I could tell my mother was feeling nervous and uncomfortable. I could tell she was unhappy. Everything felt wrong. My mother had plenty of friends whose kids were problematic like I was. Judy Collins's son killed himself. So did other friends of hers. It was the kind of thing you never got over. Mom's Italian translator had a son who killed himself; they lived in a literal castle. She was always worried about me, but, honestly, never worried enough. After I got asked to leave Dalton, I went to the day school, a small school in a church. I went there because no one else would take me.

For high school, I went to Riverdale in the Bronx. It was a long bus ride to Riverdale. I used to smoke on the school bus. Kids would ask me if I was worried about getting caught. I used to say that I never worried about getting caught because no one cared.

"Why do you need to go to rehab?" my mother asked.

"Because I'm going to die," I said.

I glanced at the driver, who was watching me in the rearview mirror.

I needed a smoke in the worst possible way. I asked the driver if I could light a cigarette.

"Just open the window," he said.

I did. I lit my cigarette. I could feel the smoke on my lips, teeth, tongue. Smoking soothed me in a way nothing else ever did.

"I think you're being overdramatic," my mom said.

"No, Mom," I replied. "I'm not."

"You're *fine*."

My mother never believed that I was a drunk. She never believed that she was one, either, always claiming that she was too famous to get sober. She would sometimes go to AA meetings, and would sometimes write about them, which you're not supposed to do—hence the "anonymous" part. She hated the whole thing. She hated the basements. She hated the people, who she believed always wanted something from her. Sometimes she would give interviews about how much she loved being sober, then she'd stop going to meetings and would promptly start drinking again, claiming she wasn't an alcoholic. This cycle repeated itself ad nauseam.

My mom wrote the novel *Any Woman's Blues* about AA, and in 1990 told the *L.A. Times*, "In my own way, I've been an addict. You cannot have been alive in the last decade without knowing someone whose life has been affected by these problems. To me, [AA] has been a very important tool, it's a self-diagnosis tool, and a real path to introspection and spirituality." Maybe Mom wasn't an alcoholic, but she did spend much of my life bouncing in and out of AA.

"Please," I said.

"Fine," she acquiesced. "But just let me go do this reading."

On November 1, 1997, I flew from LaGuardia to Minneapolis. It was raining that morning. In the lounge, I drank three vodka cranberries and took two Klonopin. I ate a bag of candy that was popular back then, Taffy-Lite. Licorice flavor. Absolutely disgusting.

On the plane I had three glasses of white wine. The wine burned my throat in that wonderful warm way wine does. I felt that calm, those fifteen minutes of calm I was always chasing.

HOW TO LOSE YOUR MOTHER

Then we landed in Minneapolis. My mom was with me. The plan was for her to drop me off at the airport and catch a flight back to New York.

We picked up my bags and went off to the arrival gate.

"But I'm going to be sober too," my mother said. She looked at me. The lady who was going to drive me to rehab was standing there, staring at both of us. "I'm going to be sober, too."

She was? I tried to hide my irritation under a blanket of drunkenness.

"I'll be sober too," she reiterated. "We'll both be sober together."

She gave me a hug.

I got into the station wagon with the elderly volunteer. We drove to Center City, Minnesota, and my mother flew back to real life. That life did not involve being sober.

I stayed at the rehab for the month of November 1997. It snowed multiple feet of snow each day. I did chores like vacuuming and mopping. I smoked lots of cigarettes. I made coffee in the coffee machine with extra packs, so it was almost undrinkably strong. I had Thanksgiving there. I appreciated the cinematic nature of Thanksgiving in rehab. I went home in December. When I got home, I had to relearn everything all over again, everything. Everything made me want to drink. But I just went to meetings and did what AA told me to do. Getting sober was worth it, and more importantly I didn't die. I've now been sober for a long time. I talk about my sobriety not because I'm so great, but because it's so meaningful in my life. I may have my problems, but being drunk now isn't one of them. My mother lost a lot of her life to drinking. Maybe most of it, actually.

Mom wasn't well, she was never well, but we always

pretended otherwise. It was easy to pretend otherwise, because she was on TV, and in magazines, and giving speeches, but inside, she was deeply, deeply unwell. And everything she did in her life—or in the part of her life when I've known her, from age thirty-seven to now—was done in the hopes of surviving her illness, which was alcoholism. And maybe even though things looked fancy on the outside, my mom was dry-rotting on the inside.

6

My life has now become the story of a little girl wearing her mother's enormous high heels through meetings with accountants and lawyers and doctors. I am talking to the movers and special fancy nursing home people who will charge lots of money for who knows what. For the last week, every day I have gone over there and sat in the weird dining room, the one I grew up sitting in. Every day I visit my parents in the apartment I grew up in. They're not children, not exactly, but they're not adults anymore either. They are like people, they look like people, but they aren't making the kind of decisions that high-, or even average-functioning people make. I will soon have to sell the apartment, and at the bottom of the New York City real estate market. I have to manage things.

I have finally made the decision to put my mother and stepfather in the World's Most Expensive Nursing Home. Like with Matt's cancer, I couldn't say the words that accurately described what was going on, so I spoke in synonyms. It wasn't a "home"; it was a "hotel." It wasn't "cancer"; it was a "mass." The surgeon, while explaining the pathology, worded it sternly: "It's a cancer." I'd always thought of myself as a very honest person, incredibly frank, but my inability to say the word "cancer," or "nursing home," indicates what a liar I am, how I have an inability to face simple facts. Mom always thought of herself as a truth teller, but the truth was that she lived in her own dreamworld, a fantasy of her own making, in which she was the one and only queen. Saying wildly inappropriate things when intoxicated does not necessarily a truth teller make. Could it be that Mom and I were actually the same?

A friend had told me about this fancy nursing home, Inspīr. I took a tour. It was a very nice place. I remembered my grandmother Eda, living in one room of her six-room apartment on Central Park West at the end of her life. For a decade, she lay in that bed in that room; for a decade Grandma was alone in that room, waiting to die. I decided this place was nicer than being alone in a room. I don't know if it was a good choice. It felt like the only choice.

I came to Mom and Ken's apartment every day with a book about the nursing home, a luxe hardcover coffee-table book with beautiful pictures of the home's five restaurants, its gym, its spa, its espresso lounge, its yoga studio, its saltwater pool. "You like to swim, right, Mom?" I'd ask. Every day, I'd sit with them in their dog-pee-smelling apartment and show them the pages of the book. Mom was impressed by the restaurants. Sometimes they seemed open to the idea of moving, and sometimes not. And just like Brigadoon, the thought would vanish and every night they'd forget the conversation. So every morning I'd have to remind them again.

I'd say happy, positive things like "It's a hotel!" and "It's like it's the Four Seasons!" And it truly *is* like the Four Seasons. And probably even more expensive. It is beautifully designed—airy and light. I said things to make myself feel better, but it wasn't clear that they knew what anything I was saying meant, and the reality of what I was doing did not change. I was putting them in a home. I was doing it because they both have dementia. I was doing it because I am a bad daughter who won't devote her life to taking care of them, the way my sister-in-law did for my in-laws. I am a bad daughter. But then again, they were terrible parents, so perhaps we're tied.

In my dark moments, I'm honest with myself. I know what I'm doing is wrong. I know they don't want to go there. I know they are not joiners. They are special. They have always thought of themselves as just a little too special to do the stuff normal people do. They have always considered themselves to be just a little too good for normal life.

Now I'm going to attempt to explain to you why I'm doing this. You're a complete stranger, but I desperately want you to know that I'm not a bad person. Or at least I'm not a bad person in *that* way. Ken had never been able to be honest with himself, which had been a huge benefit in his domestic life, given that he was the only person who was ever able to stay married to my mom. My mom, whom I adore more than a daughter has ever loved a mother, was also one of the hardest people in the world to be married to. My mom was like a movie star in her inability to not cheat and in her inability to behave normally in a marriage. How this happened, I don't know. Her parents stayed married. Her sisters stayed married. I've stayed married. But Mom could not. Mom told me that she and my father had had an open marriage. My sponsor Susan C. told me that *Mom and Ken* did, too.

I want you to empathize with my mother. Something happened to her, something in her childhood that made her disassociate. I don't know what it was. She never knew either, but whatever it was, it made it impossible for her to stay in her own body. I just don't want you, the reader, to blame her. I truly don't think any of this was her fault. Also, I want you to know that she missed so much of her life.

I don't want you to hate any of these people, but I do want to write about how bad her own parents were, and that having bad parents made her not responsible for the way she parented me. I want to make you love all of them, make them sympathetic characters. I want to explain to you how my mother was a deeply broken person who went from man to man trying to find an identity. I want to show you how she could not stop drinking because she was completely incapable of being honest with herself and others.

Listen. Erica Jong was never well. It started at a young age. My grandmother Eda was volatile and crazy. She broke dishes and screamed at everyone and was just furious that she wasn't a famous painter. I have mentioned that Eda ripped her clothing off on the bus. Eda was the queen of the public scene. Later my mother made scenes like that. Later my mother would scream in the street and act out on the bus (though my mother has never been one for public transportation).

Grandma was also a terrible drunk. She loved vodka. "*Vod*ka," she'd say with her fancy, affected Mid-Atlantic accent. She was born in London, in the slums of London, but London nevertheless. They were climbers, my mother's family. If you asked, Mom would say they were "bohemians." Grandma had been a painter and Grandpa was a drummer. But they weren't really bohemians—they were Jews trying to create themselves again in this brave new world. My grandfather was born in the slums, too—of Brooklyn. Both of my mother's parents came to Manhattan to escape poverty.

HOW TO LOSE YOUR MOTHER

My mother's childhood, in Manhattan of the 1940s and 1950s, was a time of incredible social mobility. Most of the kids Mom grew up with on the Upper West Side were also the children of Jewish immigrants. They went to very good public schools and spent their afternoons in the library or at the movies or in the park. She used to say that when she was a kid the city was dirty and poor, but also filled with possibilities. She described men sitting on wooden crates on Columbus Avenue, playing cards. People were poor, but there was a sense anything could happen, and often it did. Those kids grew up to run movie studios and the Federal Reserve. They went on to run the world. Their grandfathers had been merchants and tailors, and in half a generation they'd become masters of the universe. It was hard to come from that world and not think absolutely anything was possible.

I took my friend Taffy Brodesser-Akner to see Mom in her apartment. Taffy is the author of the novel *Fleishman Is in Trouble*, and she wrote the amazing television adaptation, too. She had been hired to write a movie about my mother, which is how we became friends. Taffy is probably more famous now than Erica Jong is, which adds an odd dynamic. Taffy's movie is the story of Mom's disastrous lawsuit against Columbia Pictures and the late producer Julia Phillips. My mother, back when she was still able to talk about such high-flying topics, claimed that the lawsuit, to regain the film rights to *Fear of Flying*, was the biggest mistake she ever made. The lawsuit, which she lost, destroyed her career. She'd always believed that, and she was probably at least a little bit right. In her memoir *You'll Never Eat Lunch in This Town Again*, Phillips wrote that my mother looked like Miss Piggy.

Taffy has read all the court records and testimonies, plus the news coverage, and talked to everyone she could—well, everyone who's still alive, which is arguably not that many people—about the debacle with Columbia Pictures. Taffy has read through the Erica Jong Archive, which is housed at Columbia University. Taffy has seen Mom's datebooks from the seventies. Taffy has read *Fear of Flying* about ten thousand times. Taffy loves Mom in a way that I wish I did.

"It wasn't your fault," Taffy said to Mom. She was trying to make her feel better about suing Columbia Pictures. "You were given bad advice. You had a producer who was volatile and unpredictable and disrespectful. You never stood a chance." Taffy was trying to tell her how to let herself off the hook for this thing that happened so long ago—how so many people made bad or pernicious decisions that it really didn't matter. Hollywood is a company town where the house always wins, and an Upper West Side writer cannot come in and sue Columbia Pictures and hope that victory awaits her.

But Mom was right. Suing Columbia Pictures probably *did* ruin her career.

"They were all taking advantage of you," Taffy said. Also true.

Taffy and I stayed for a few hours. Mom was dirty. The weekend aide seemed kind of nuts. For a second, it occurred to me that the weekend aide might want to poison Mom and Ken. I knew this was crazy, but I didn't eat any of the food there anyway.

Today was move-in day. My sister-in-law took their poodles with her to her house in the country, where they'll live with a giant rescue bichon frise named Choppy who has a forty-pound head. My parents hadn't seemed to notice that their dogs were gone.

"We gave you power of attorney, and you put us in a home,"

Mom said, as we arrived at the World's Most Expensive Nursing Home.

This was, on the face of it, true.

Basically, the whole thing was reverse summer-camp drop-off. You lied to your parents just like you lied to your kids. But with the kids, you knew that they were going for a short period of time. With the parents, they were going forever. With the kids, you knew you were doing something for their own good; with the parents you were not so sure. Also, with the kids, you were pretty confident that they weren't going to die there. With your parents, you knew they were.

A couple of days later, I called my dad, my one remaining parent. I was in a taxi heading to CNN, to do a late-night panel. I told him that Mom wasn't dead yet but that she wasn't exactly in there anymore. I told him that all she did was sleep and drink. I told him how guilty I felt. I said that I shouldn't be at the CNN studios. Wherever I was, I felt I should have been somewhere else. I should have been spending more time with my kids, with my parents, with my dogs, with my cancerous husband.

My dad tried to reassure me in his own peculiar, fucked-up way.

"You know," he said, "when you were a little girl, the nanny and I used to try and get your mom to spend time with you. We tried to get her to spend just *an hour a day* with you."

This admission made me feel *so* great.

"And she couldn't do it," my dad said. "She couldn't even spend *one hour* with you. The most she could do was half an hour."

Now maybe my father was trying to use this knowledge as a way to make me feel less guilty about putting her in a home. Because when I go to visit her, she is always crying. She wasn't a crier when I was a child, but she cries a lot now. Everyone who works there is worried. They are worried about Mom. They are worried about the crying, but they are really, *really* worried about the drinking. And the more she drinks, the more she cries. (And the more she cries, the more she drinks.)

One of the first things the fancy nursing home did was set my mom and Ken up with their pot doc. They thought it would help with their anxiety. The pot doc was a short man with very blue eyes. Weirdly, he grew up on the Upper West Side with my dad. We were all in my mom's strange new living room—the pot doc, Mom, Ken, and my mom's sister. I was sitting on the floor. My aunt has MS. When the doctor tried to explain the benefits of pot to my mom, she started crying. Then she started complaining about her parents. She said she wouldn't be the way she was if it weren't for her parents' drinking.

My aunt bristled at the suggestion that Grandma and Grandpa were alcoholics.

"They *always* drank," Mom said. I really hated seeing her cry. It was very upsetting to me. "Mother *and* Daddy were big drinkers."

My aunt interrupted. "No, no. Not Daddy."

Who cares, I said to myself. *Who the actual fuck cares?* They've been dead for more than a decade. No one cares.

"Daddy *never* drank," my aunt added.

As someone who has been sober for far longer than I was an addict, I will submit that there is something super annoying about the phenomenon of alcoholics and their families pretending they're not alcoholics. So many people die of alcoholism, but instead of using those deaths as a grim cautionary tale, we pretend that a thirty-eight-year-old just didn't get up one morning. More often than not, they died of alcoholism. I truly believe that if we were honest about our addictions, many more of us would get sober, and far fewer of us would die. I never knew people could get sober as teenagers and stay sober. I didn't know that was something that could happen until I did it. I always think that if one person understands they can remain sober because they saw me do it, then it's all worth it. I brag about my alcoholism, and my sobriety. I do it because I think it can help people, but if nothing else, it helps *me*. It helps me stay sober.

"I could never get sober," my mother said. She was still crying. "Everyone in AA just wanted to give me their manuscripts. Everyone just wanted help getting an agent."

Ah, yes. The old I'm Too Famous to Get Sober excuse. Well, I'm a prominent person in the world now, too. I mean, I had gotten a little bit famous. Not really *famous* famous, just *recognized*, and just in, you know, certain places. It was a bit like my mom's fame at the end, not at the beginning when she was on the cover of national magazines. Like when people sort of give me the once-over, wondering if, or how, they know me.

"Actually, *I'm* on TV all the time," I said.

I hate saying stuff about myself—it's so insecure and defensive—but I want to crush my mother's stupid notion that she's too "important" for AA. My mother is barely in there, but I'm still fighting with her.

"And *I'm* fine using AA," I add.

But because this is my family, no one listened to me. They just kept talking over me—and one another. Yet somehow, I'm now the boss of everyone, the power of attorney, the functional one.

The pot doctor gave both my mother and stepfather pot pills. It's now abundantly clear that anyone can get pot for anything these days. Even though I went for much, much harder stuff than pot when I was an addict, this is just at the edge of my comfort zone.

After about an hour, I had the thrilling observation I could just leave.

So I did.

Later, my aunt called me to say that she didn't think my mom should be doing pot. She thought there were other solutions.

"You know," she added, "my friend Sharon quit her job at *The New York Times* to take care of *her* mother."

I told my aunt that I would be delighted if her friend Sharon would like to have my mother and stepfather live with her and her mother.

I kept getting calls. This time from my godmother, Gerri. She wanted me to know that she was worried about how out-of-it my mother is. I reminded her that my mother has dementia.

Gerri lets it be known (as has my aunt, and my mom's assistant) that she wants me to move Mom back to her own apartment—which smelled like pee (both dog and human), which had a bed with shit (dog or human?) in it, where they were in danger every day.

I am furious with all of them.

When I was growing up, my mother and Ken collected rare books. They'd always lecture me about their enormous value. He bought her first editions of lots of famous books. They were delighted by their collection.

Here is a typical scene from my young adulthood:

"Moll," Ken would say, "I bought your mother a copy of *Ulysses*."

"Okay," I would say. I hadn't read *Ulysses*. I didn't care.

"It's a *first edition*," Ken would add.

"Okay," I would say, fiddling with my phone.

My mother would emerge from elsewhere in their apartment and join in the conversation.

"You *know*," she would say. She was still youngish then, and I was in my twenties. "Someday all these books will be *yours*. My collection! Someday all the rare books Ken and I bought each other will be yours, and they'll be wildly valuable, and you'll *treasure* them."

Now I was trying to sell it all. While I'd been trying to save some of their stuff, I decided to sell the books. Sotheby's came to the apartment for an appraisal. They seemed interested at first, but somewhere along the way, they changed their minds. I decided to call Doyle, an auction house several rungs down the auction-house hierarchy from Sotheby's.

It was one of those weird days when it was March but still freezing. I was wearing a heavy coat and I was in a taxi, taking a kid to therapy. The man from Doyle was weird and suspicious on the phone.

"Why are you selling these books *now*?" he asked skeptically.

I sensibly explained that I didn't think they'd do well in storage, and I was not convinced that they'd increase in value.

He seemed unconvinced. He seemed to think I was some kind of monster.

I went on to explain that my parents were no longer in their apartment—they were in a nursing home and that we needed to downsize.

While I was in the waiting room at the therapist's office, I got a call from Matt's doctor. She wanted to talk to us about his

PET scan. This is never good. We conferenced Matt in.

Dr. O'Reilly was halting. These doctors are always halting when they have something terrible to tell you.

"The PET scan lit up at the liver," she said.

I looked around the waiting room. I was trying to keep from crying, again. What happens to the tears you never cry? Do they get reabsorbed into you, or do they linger? Do those uncried tears continue to travel around your body, all pain, all sadness?

7

Part of taking over my parents' ever-dwindling estate was reckoning with the fact that my mother and stepfather lived way beyond their means. I grew up thinking we were rich. I flew on the Concorde, for example, though often it was paid for by my mom's work. I stayed in five-star hotels. I attended private schools. We lived in that haunted townhouse. I believed, because of the way my mother spent money, that we were incredibly wealthy. My stepfather had a sailboat and small plane. My parents drove luxury cars. My mother had an enormous emerald ring. What I had always feared—and, frankly, suspected—now turned out to be true: they had spent every cent they had, and then some. And now the bill had come due. Someone had to sell the apartment, clean up everything, fire the housekeeper, the assistants. And that someone was good old me. When I did drugs, I was the kind of addict who would go through your medicine cabinet. I am not that kid anymore. Now I'm the squarest, sanest, most responsible member of the family. Now I'm the one who has to fire the housekeeper.

Maria is from Mexico. My parents hired her as their housekeeper when I was in my twenties. She had one of those lives you see in movies. And I had to tell her that we couldn't afford her anymore. She wept. I wept. I never thought I would, or could, make someone cry like that.

We were standing in my mother's office in their empty apartment. Her green carpet was covered in stains.

"Your mother promised she would take care of me," Maria said through tears.

The funny thing was that my mother told me the same thing. She always told me that I was going to inherit millions of dollars. I feel ungrateful and spoiled and victim-y for even bringing this up, but every chance she ever had, my mother would tell me about all the money I was going to inherit. While I always thought we were rich, like very rich, the truth was that they could barely be bothered to make a will. And this is fine. No one is entitled to anything. But the point is that they turned out to be exactly who I always thought they were.

"But your mother always told me that the art on the walls is worth millions of dollars," Maria said.

I looked around. Some of the art was indeed valuable, but a lot of it, like the Larry Rivers, the Red Grooms, the stuff that might have been very popular in the eighties and nineties, was now wildly out of fashion. You always read about the artists who become wealthy and popular, but most artists just disappear. Just like most writers. There's no permanence to anything.

I apologized profusely. I handed Maria what I thought of as an enormous check. But I wasn't sorry, I was furious, though I shouldn't have been. People always make promises they can't or don't have any intention of keeping.

"It's not enough," she said. "New York is very expensive."

*

HOW TO LOSE YOUR MOTHER

I went to visit my parents at the nursing home. My younger son met me in the lobby. We took the elevator up to the seventh floor.

We opened the door to their apartment. Mom was in a state—far more disheveled, and panicked, than usual.

"Will I die here? In *two rooms*? I don't want to die in two rooms."

We went over to the dining table. I wanted to have a reasonable conversation.

"We could keep this as a country house," my stepfather said helpfully, from the sofa.

I was so tired. We were all so tired. My brain was so scrambled from everything. My brain was so scrambled from politics, from Twitter. My brain was so scrambled from my year of unfathomable loss. My brain was so scrambled that I worried I was becoming my mother.

"Just stay here for today," I said.

They were unsatisfied. My stepfather asked me if I fired the housekeeper. I told him I did.

He said, "She keeps a good kitchen."

My phone rang. My beloved godmother, Gerri. I answered on speaker. Mom didn't seem to remember who Gerri was. Gerri stated that she had some bad news.

"I have blood cancer," she said.

My mom was silent. She and my stepfather had no clue about what was happening in the real world, in the normal nondemented world. I could feel tears building up behind my eyes.

"I can't live forever," Gerri, ever the stoic, said. "Oh well."

The last time we'd spoken, I'd yelled at Gerri in fury for suggesting that I move Mom out of the nursing home. I now apologized for yelling at her then. I told her that I was so incredibly sorry. We ended the call. I felt like throwing up. Mom looked at me in a daze.

"Mom," I said, "Gerri is dying."

Mom didn't seem to understand. Ken also could not process the information.

Everyone was dying. Everyone was always dying, all the time. For my whole life, no one ever died, and now everyone was dying all around me.

I went home to Matt. We had a video appointment with the oncologist. We took the call in the bedroom so the children couldn't hear. Our bedroom is small and square, with two windows. The late afternoon sun streamed in through the window, making patterns on the wood floor. It was that kind of sharp afternoon light that you can see the dust in. We bought this apartment when I was pregnant with my twins. Those twins are now fifteen years old. We've had trouble trying to figure out what the children should know and what they shouldn't know. We are puzzled. I've always thought of myself as a relatively good parent, but now I'm not so sure.

The doctor appeared on the screen of Matt's computer. She was not as cheerful as she once had been. That flush of optimism was gone.

"Matt could live decades," she said.

But what we noticed was that the doctor was no longer talking about a cure. This is no longer curative.

We tried to pin her down on odds. We asked her, in a million different ways, what his chances were. She wouldn't answer.

"The future is uncertain for all of us," she said.

*

HOW TO LOSE YOUR MOTHER

Whenever my mother was in danger of feeling anything, she would travel. It was now spring break, though I had already stopped existing in the normal waves of domestic life. I decided to take the children to L.A. My dad is there, and so is his son, my half brother. I decided that taking the children on a normal spring break vacation would be good for the children and good for me. I've started to think of myself as just a little bit cursed. I was now starting to get worried for the people around me. Was I some kind of death amulet, a Horcrux? Was I a human Chernobyl? Did the people around me simply fall ill and die? Was it all somehow my fault? Was there something I was inadvertently doing to cause all this chaos and suffering?

We had tickets on a very early Saturday flight. Don't ask me why I thought it was a good idea to book this time. Although I was bleary-eyed from lack of sleep, I liked that we were going on a trip like a normal family in which the father is not maybe probably possibly dying. Of course, Matt wasn't coming with us, so we were a normal family without a father. A few days before, Matt's ninety-one-year-old father had been hospitalized. He was still in the hospital.

At JFK, I ran into lots of people I knew. A cousin of Matt's, an MSNBC host, a friend of my son's. People asked me where Matt was. I told them he had to catch up on work. I didn't tell them that he was dying, or maybe dying, or that maybe he could outrun the cancer.

I listened to *The Year of Magical Thinking* on the plane. I start thinking about Joan Didion. When Sotheby's first came to my parents' apartment, they said that perhaps they'd do an auction with my mother's stuff, just as they'd done with Joan Didion. But then they apparently decided that Mom was not good enough for

Sotheby's. And all the priceless books turned out not to be so priceless after all. So I took everything to Doyle. The Doyle guy wasn't the weird, hostile person I'd spoken with on the phone; this other guy was extremely nice, and very young, and made me feel better about the fact that my mother isn't as famous as Joan. I knew Joan's daughter, Quintana, fairly well, and she wasn't a particularly happy person. Actually, she was miserable. And she died very young.

But Joan had the advantage of not just writing about herself, and about being interested in other things, which I guess is why they were able to sell her sunglasses for more than a hundred thousand dollars. Also, Joan was very thin and glamorous. Joan wrote better than Mom, but that does not necessarily matter when it comes to writer-fame, though perhaps in this case it does.

As we were getting seated on the plane, Matt texted me. We were a normal family where the father didn't come along because he still had a surgical drain because he'd recently had numerous organs removed.

The text read: "there's blood in the drain."

I looked at the text bleary-eyed.

"I don't understand," I typed.

He texted: "I'm going to get a CAT scan."

I asked him if I should get off the plane and come home.

Then I just saw the dots. Those infernal dots. He was writing. People were still coming onto the plane.

"Just go," Matt typed.

Matt's sister couldn't come to be with him because she was in the hospital with their father, which meant Matt would have to have the procedure alone.

I was so tired and sad I felt like I was going to die. But we stayed on the plane. Was this the right thing to do?

I started listening to *The Year of Magical Thinking* again: "The future always looks good in the golden land, because no one remembers the past."

I thought about Didion and the golden land. Maybe I'd have eight days of reprieve from the grimness of my current situation. Of course, my trip was escapism. Of course it was. I was hoping to forget the real world, to enter some kind of place in the space-time continuum where mesoscopic bits of cancer weren't floating around Matt's body, trying to find an organ to grow in. At a recent doctor's appointment, I had asked Matt if he wanted to go back in time.

"That's not how string theory works," Matt had said.

"Yes, it is," I had said. "It means that other times are going on at the same time."

"Not really," he had replied. "But with all this stuff, you have to decide what you believe and what you don't believe."

I am not immune to the siren's song of the West Coast, the skyline of palm trees and blurry blue sky. I am not immune to the charm of its bungalows and citrus fruit. I was listening to Joan Didion, weird Joan—so fancy, so conservative. I kept telling myself that I am not someone who lives on the West Coast. I am a New Yorker, tried and true. But now I play this weird game where I wonder what will happen when Matt dies. Not *if*, but *when*. Maybe the Widow Jong-Fast, still in her forties, will move to California. But I can't think like that, I tell myself, I can't think like that. This isn't about me. I am not Erica Jong. Not everything is about me.

You have to decide what you believe and what you don't believe.

Did I mention I used to hate flying? Saying I hated flying is actually kind of wrong. I didn't hate flying. I was obsessed with my hatred of flying: with worrying about flying, worrying about turbulence, worrying about weather. I was obsessed with every little noise the plane made. I stared at maps I didn't know how to read.

I came by my fear of flying honestly. Mom was afraid of flying, despite the fact that she grew up on an airplane. Her father, Seymour Mann, was an importer. Being an "importer" is one of those jobs that no longer exists. His entire job was fly to Japan, find cheap stuff, buy it, bring it back, and sell it for an enormous markup. His job was basically being a shopper. My grandfather didn't speak Japanese or have great taste or anything; his main talent was that he could get on a plane in the 1950s and fly to Japan. The planes were not great then. Nor were the flight schedules. My grandfather would be gone for months and months. He would be gone for so long that my grandmother decided that he had another family in Japan, so she started going on these trips with him. My mother and her two sisters would be left with my grandmother's father's papa. (I guess that makes him my great-great-grandfather?) Papa and Mama were from the old country (Russia, Ukraine—or some country between the two that doesn't exist anymore and maybe never ever did). They were big worriers. They believed that pretty much everything would kill you. They didn't let Mom ride a bike. They didn't let Mom roller-skate. They wanted to keep her in Bubble Wrap. They always made her feel like she was in danger. Whatever happened there laid the groundwork for her pathological fear of flying.

And the alcohol made both my mother and grandmother wildly irrational. They became deeply superstitious. They got involved in crystals. Every flight they took became some kind of weird cultist ritual. They would do this kind of chant before they stepped onto the plane. Between them and my nanny Margaret, who believed she could predict the future because she'd had dreams right before her baby and her husband died, it's amazing I'm as rational as I am. (Not that I'm rational.)

"Sunny" California was not sunny during this particular spring break. L.A. was cold. It rained every day. We stayed at the Beverly Hills Hotel, where my mother and I lived for a month in the eighties when the pilot for her TV show was being shot. This is also the place where my father's parents used to live—now that enormous parking structure behind the hotel. The kids had stayed here before. One trip—with my mother, of course—was particularly memorable. When they were small, Matt and I didn't have money for travel, so my mom would take us on work trips with her. Once she put us up with her at the hallowed Beverly Hills Hotel. The first night we were there, she went out to dinner with, supposedly, a famous producer. This supposedly famous producer wanted to make a movie of *Fear of Flying*. I'd been hearing this my whole life—everyone always wanted to make a movie of *Fear of Flying*, except they didn't really want to, or if they did, the deal always fell apart, like most things in Hollywood.

Mom was very excited about the trip, about the dinner. She believed this would finally be the moment she would get what she so richly deserved. Mom always felt she hadn't gotten the recognition she was entitled to, despite everything, despite her success, despite her luck. She was always felt it wasn't fair.

I wasn't at the dinner. She came back to the hotel after midnight. I was in the room next door with my kids. She knocked on the door. I opened it and there she stood, with a huge bruise on her thigh. I could smell white wine on her breath.

I asked her if she was okay. I knew she was not okay.

"I fell," she said.

She lifted her skirt to show me more of the bruise on her thigh.

"These damn shoes," she said.

"Mom," I said. I inhaled. "It's not the shoes. You're drunk."

"I *just* had wine." Mom truly believed that wine was nothing more potent than Mott's Apple Juice.

I brought her back to her room and laid her down in her bed, in the way a million daughters of alcoholic mothers have before me.

"I just had wine," she repeated.

I tucked her into the sheets, the thick, clean, white sheets.

"I just had wine," she said again.

The following morning, I took the children to the pool at the hotel. We'd gotten a cabana. The kids ate French fries, and played video games, and jumped into the pool. It was perfect, one of those moments when L.A. lived up to your expectations of it. Mom came down to the pool later in the day. I had been trying to go to an AA meeting every day and I needed one now. The previous night's daughter-of-an-alcoholic reprisal of my childhood had made me crunchy and dry-drunkish. I needed a meeting or I was going to yell at everyone. AA meetings kept me sane and continue to.

Mom didn't look so great. I asked her if she was okay.

"The hotel doctor said I was fine."

Mom was always seeing hotel doctors for falls and bumps. I'll bet that most people don't even know that hotels *have* doctors. Well, they do, and Erica Jong had personal relationships with various doctors at various hotels. A few years before, she'd become good friends with a hotel doctor who took care of her after she'd hit her head on the room safe.

"He said I should drink some sangria by the pool and take it easy," she said.

I tried not to hear what she was saying. Mom had a shrink, a very old shrink, who didn't believe she was an alcoholic. The shrink was obsessed with Mom and seemed to believe that a little white wine was good for her. Sometimes Mom and I would have joint sessions and the shrink would imply (none too subtly) that I was too sensitive to alcoholism because I was sober. I asked her if it was all right if I went to my AA meeting. I asked her if she could watch the kids.

"It will be like for an hour and a half. The meeting starts at 12:00 and ends at 1:00. I'll be back by 1:30. Possible?"

"Of course," she said.

I should have told her not to drink. I should have told her that she needed to be sober, I should have begged her to stay sober.

When I returned to the hotel an hour and a half later, Mom was passed out on a lounge chair in the cabana. There was a half-empty pitcher of sangria. She looked as if she were dead. It was the state I often found her in when I was a kid and I'd come in to give her a kiss before I went to sleep. She would still have on the dress she'd worn to dinner.

My older son, who was then eleven, looked up from his video game.

"We think Grandma is dead," he said, and went back to the game.

My daughter, who was seven, looked up from her iPad. She had a different take on Grandma's condition.

"Grandma's not dead," she said. "She's still breathing."

I apologized to my kids for leaving them alone with my mother. I had rarely done it before. Not that she had offered—she was never exactly one of those sweet little selfless grannies who love to chip in with babysitting. It turned out she was exactly the same with her grandchildren as she'd been with me: gushing, lavish in her gifts, extravagant in her praise, and never present. I told them I would never leave them alone with her again.

No one was hurt. No one drowned, although they absolutely could have. And it would have been my fault. I knew the stakes. I knew what could happen. I had tried to protect my children from my mother's alcoholism, but I had failed.

In L.A., I had lunch with my half-brother and his boss at a Del Frisco's in the Westfield Century City Mall. It was still raining because it rained six out of the eight days we were in Los Angeles. Of course it did. I had to come to L.A. to get away from the rain in my life, but you can't escape the rain, you can never escape the rain.

Matt texted me during lunch: "Surgeon not as optimistic about my runway as oncologist."

I thought about what the word "runway" means. It meant, in this context, how long he'll live. I thought about runways, and about the length of runways. The runways at LaGuardia are short, which is why if you want to fly a long distance on a big plane, you need to schlep all the way out to JFK.

I texted Matt that I would call him after lunch. The old feeling of doom was back, that feeling of tragedy and catastrophe that liked to sit right on my shoulder. Another text from him after lunch, as I was walking my meal off at the mall:

"This surgeon doesn't know how long I have."

HOW TO LOSE YOUR MOTHER

We have conversations like this now. Conversations people have in bad TV movies, conversations that don't seem like things real people say to each other. And all I can do is lie.

"It's going to be okay."

My dad and stepmom took the children to Disneyland. I saw my friend Dana for dinner. She is a fifty-five-year-old widow. I hugged her and considered the calculus of our lives. Luck. What is luck? Sometimes, we have luck, and sometimes we just don't. Dana buried Chuck during the pandemic. Chuck died of cancer. He had been sick for a long time. Years. Dana drove him to doctors' appointments and surgery. Eventually, there was nothing the doctors could do, and Chuck died. Dana survived. Chuck and Dana were at my wedding to Matt. It is now twenty years later. Dana told me things I should be doing now that I'm a member of the Wives of Cancer-Husbands Club, but I didn't listen. She wanted me to join a Wives of Cancer-Husbands support group. I nodded, pretending I would join, but I won't. I'm only forty-four years old. I don't want to be a widow or a potential widow or someone auditioning for the role of widow. I want to be normal. A normal person with a normal life.

Dana said she's happy now. She has a new boyfriend who writes for the *L.A. Times*.

I promised myself I would never get divorced. I promised myself that my children would always have two parents. I promised myself that, but much of what happens in our lives isn't up to us.

"We continue on," Dana said.

Was I even sure that I *could* continue?

"Yes," I said. "We do."

8

I started to notice the bags under my eyes around the time Matt got diagnosed. That's the thing about getting older, you get little peeks into it. It happens slowly, then quickly. Your body unravels like a loose-knit sweater. One day there's a moth hole, and the next day you're wondering how much a neck lift would cost and where you would hide out for a few weeks while you recover. My nanny Margaret would sometimes muse to me about what it meant to get older (this was before I got into drugs and decided I'd never have to worry about getting old). She'd say, "I'm proud of every wrinkle I have, I've earned them. I would never try to get rid of them." Meanwhile, my mom would be at a spa trying to outrun the clock.

I'd always prided myself on not being vain. I'd never been a beauty—not unattractive, but not a beauty, never ever, which, in my mind, made me depend on my wits, on my sense of humor. I wouldn't be like all those women mourning their lost beauty, never able to make sense of the cruel ravages of time.

I was sitting at my desk looking out at the cool sunny April day. My mother and stepfather now lived together in two rooms. My mother napped and drank wine at lunch and dinner and took pot pills. I was just a few blocks away at my desk, trying to work.

I had moved them into a nursing home because there were no better options.

There was something wrong on the puppy's blood tests. I cried on the phone with the vet. Since January, when Matt got diagnosed with the mass, I've had this suspicion that if I start crying, I might not be able to stop. I just have so much to cry about that my tears will overwhelm me and perhaps I'll drown. Not that this is even the worst outcome, but I do want someone to be on this planet for my children.

In the car on the way to *Morning Joe*, I cried three times, because I knew that Matt was dying, and I was not. Then I talked to my friend Jon, who is a straight-news journalist. I called him because I wanted to talk to someone before I did live TV, to make sure I was awake enough not to sound like a complete idiot. I hadn't been sleeping incredibly well since January.

Jon said, "Every marriage has a million unspoken resentments."

He was, of course, right. Anyone who has been married a long time knows this . . . but can you admit it if your spouse is sick? How can you be mad at someone who is dying? How can normal life proceed?

And then there was my mother.

She needed to have an MRI. We could tell there was something really wrong with her, wronger than her usual dementia-wrong. She was now dizzy all the time. She couldn't remember what she'd ordered at the restaurant in the nursing home even a minute after she'd placed the order.

I met my mom and her assistant in the waiting room at the doctor's office. She and Ken no longer worked, but they each still had an assistant. I will need to fire them, just as I have fired Maria.

I don't even have an assistant, and I have a job. I have more than one job, in fact. More than two, possibly even more than three.

Mom was extremely agitated.

"You okay?" I asked.

"I'm *not* going in there," she said. "It's too small. It's too tight. I don't want them to look at my brain. My brain is happy. My brain doesn't need anyone looking into it. My brain is *fine*."

I explained that there was something wrong with her brain, and that the doctors had to take a look inside it. I now speak to her as if she's a child.

"My brain is happy," she said again. "There is *nothing* wrong with my brain." She's like a child, but then again, she's always been kind of like a child. "And what if something happens and I never write again?"

When I was growing up, "never writing again" was one of my mom's central anxieties. She was always worried that it might finally hit her, that all her writing ambition and ability would be drained from her. She would be permanently blocked. Anytime something bad—or good—happened—she would panic that she would never write again. I should add that she never worried about the *quality* of her writing; but instead that the *drive* itself might somehow be taken from her—by feeling too comfortable, or too uncomfortable. I reassured her that everything would be okay during the MRI scan. It was, and the whole thing was over very quickly.

After the appointment, we stood on Seventy-Second Street, waiting for the car. She was so dizzy that she had to sit on a bench. Someone came by and recognized us. I was mortified. The car came and we went back to the nursing home she hated.

And then, in the car, she said the most extraordinary thing.

"I need a glass of wine because I'm a drunk."

So many years of telling her I thought she was an alcoholic. So many years of telling her she should stop drinking. So many years of begging my stepdad to help her get sober. And now when there was nothing for her to lose, she could finally be honest that she's a drunk. It was just like many times I tried to get my mom to quit diet pills. She was always trying to lose weight. She never actually needed to lose weight. I'd always thought that maybe she just loved the pills.

Needless to say, I spent a lot of time in my childhood in therapy. I had a shrink. My mom had a shrink. We did meetings with both our shrinks. When I was a kid, Mom had a celebrity shrink for me. Her name was Mildred Newman, and supposedly Mike Nichols and Nora Ephron were patients. She wrote a book called *How to Be Your Own Best Friend* and much of her therapeutic practice involved collecting celebrities in her East Side penthouse to do group therapy. I loved her because she gave me cookies.

One day when I was maybe eleven or twelve, Mildred cooked up this idea that I was finally going to beg my mother to stop taking diet pills. Many people in my life seemed to believe that, because my mother loved me so much (or, more precisely, because she always talked about how much she loved me), if she could just see how her drug-taking and drinking were affecting me, she would stop. Even when I was a little kid, I knew that it took a lot more than this to stop addictive behavior.

One day after school, my mom and I were in this shrink's office, sitting side by side on the sofa. Yes, there were cookies. Yes, I was eating them. I was also crying.

"Tell your mother how you feel when she's on diet pills, Molly," Dr. Newman said. She wore these amazing muumuus and always had on lots of jewelry.

Anytime Mom wanted to lose weight she would go back on diet pills. Diet pills completely changed her personality and made her delightfully manic. All of a sudden, my very removed, very busy mother would be game for anything. She would take me out shopping or out on a drive, but the problem was that the diet pills made her absolutely unhinged. I remember more than a few instances of her going off the road or running into something. None of the accidents were on purpose, I think.

At that moment in Dr. Newman's office, my mother was actually holding a Baggie of diet pills. I tried to pull the pill-Baggie from her hand.

"I feel *terrible* when you're on diet pills," I said. Little did I know that a few years later, I would have a diet-pill addiction of my own.

Mom started crying.

"I'm sorry, darling," she said through tears. "I'll stop. I promise I'll stop."

She would always say that when confronted with her addiction. And being the addict she was, she would always just keep on drinking. I was a little child, so I was dependent on her—one of the things about being dependent on someone who was constitutionally incapable of being honest with herself was that she was also constitutionally incapable of being honest with me.

I looked over at Dr. Newman.

"Can we be done now?" I begged Dr. Newman. The thing that I knew even then was that there was no way I would ever be able to get my mom to stop taking pills or to stop drinking. (It is possible that Dr. Newman was not the best shrink in the world.)

"Just tell her how you *feel*," Dr. Newman said.

It's more than thirty years later, and I still find that question absolutely unanswerable. *How do I feel?*

I feel that this is wasting my time.

I feel that my mother will never stop being an addict.

Also, I felt that we spent a lot of time talking to people who made money off our problems. And no one ever got better.

Years later, when I was sixteen or seventeen, we were on vacation in Italy. Mom was driving. My friend Amy was with us. Mom, hopped up on her beloved diet pills, drove right into a stone wall and nearly hit a man—a farmer who was out on a walk. The farmer was unhurt, but was understandably furious, and I remember thinking, *My mother is a dangerous person. My mother is going to end up killing someone. And that someone could be me.* (Not that I, the professional delusion-respecter, ever stopped riding with her.)

My mother was a bad driver, like Jordan Baker. I happened to be reading *The Great Gatsby*, on that trip to Italy. Jordan reproaches Nick: "'You said a bad driver was only safe until she met another bad driver? Well, I met another bad driver, didn't I? I mean it was careless of me to make such a wrong guess. I thought you were rather an honest, straightforward person. I thought it was your secret pride.'"

It took two careless people to cause an accident. Did this mean, given that our life was one big slow-motion accident, that I was a bad driver, too?

The results from the MRI came back. No plaque. No Alzheimer's. She was just demented. Just your normal old garden-variety late-stage-alcoholic demented.

*

When I first met Matt, I told him my mother was an alcoholic, but he didn't really believe me. I would try to tell him that every night when she was at home, I'd find her passed out on the bed, eye makeup everywhere, lipstick smeared on the coverlet. But I was only twenty-three, and he thought I was being a touch hyperbolic. Besides, *I* had been the one who needed to get sober. And, despite bouncing in and out of recovery much of her life, and writing the novel *Any Woman's Blues* about AA, most people thought my mom was fine because she was successful. It was at my first cousin's wedding when he understood that what I'd told him about my mother wasn't an exaggeration.

I got pregnant when Matt and I were engaged. My mom wasn't the kind of mother who even particularly wanted me to get married, and I didn't know how she'd react to either piece of the news. We asked them to dinner. Before dinner, I vomited in their bathroom. At the restaurant, we told them we were engaged, but the big news was still to come.

"I think I might be pregnant," I said.

"That's *wonderful* news," my mother exclaimed.

Ken smiled.

"This is the *greatest* thing to happen!" she added. "A grandchild! *Wonderful!*"

I was completely freaked out that I was ruining my life. But I was going to have this child.

My feminist mother seemed elated. So maybe I *wasn't* going to ruin my life after all? Her responses to things were often so unpredictable. But one of the great things about my mom was that she was always so proud of me, always so delighted by everything I did. I guess I had thought that she was going to have some sort of insane drunken response. She could easily have given an intoxicated speech about the wonders of her own pregnancy with me . . . or just as likely she might launch into a crazy sermon about how children ruin a woman's career. Instead, Mom was so supportive, so thrilled for me.

I thought about what kind of grandmother she would make. Would she be glamorous, distracted, detached, just as she'd been with me? Or would she be maybe a little less glamorous, but more engaged, more present? She had never been able to mother me, but now maybe she would be able to grandmother my child?

Matt and I had a very short engagement. We got married a few months later. Later that fall, he and I were in a hotel in Vermont for my cousin's wedding. I was very fat already. I had bought a stretchy dress. I had just put the dress on and was looking at myself in the mirror. I could see that besides gaining weight in my stomach, which hopefully was at least some percentage baby, I had also gained a ton of weight in my thighs.

I had a bad feeling about tonight.

"She's going to get drunk and make an insane speech," I told Matt.

He is one of these people who delights in denial. This is not a criticism. It is, if anything, a compliment.

"I don't know why you're freaking out so much," he said. "I'm sure it's going to be fine."

But I knew that it would not be fine. If a person could die of embarrassment, my mother would have killed me a long time ago. She could not *not* drink, and once she started drinking, she started toasting. I never ever went to a wedding or to a bar mitzvah or to a party or to anything with my mother in which she didn't get very drunk, then grab the microphone and give a toast. It always started off seeming as if it might be okay, but then the situation would develop into a high crazy. I don't know if she always had this problem, or she just got it from being famous, but my mom was obsessed with saying exactly what you knew you weren't supposed to say. If someone had a birthmark, or was very fat or something, she would absolutely say something about it. It was like some kind of Tourette's syndrome. I got very used to apologizing for her. I became a brilliant apologizer. I was like the Sun Tzu of apologizing.

Matt did not know what it was like. He didn't understand the entitlement that came to my mother from her fame. She really truly believed that everyone *wanted* her to speak. On some level, I think she thought that people would be disappointed if she didn't speak.

We got to the wedding reception. I had this rash that made my whole enormous belly itch like crazy. I tried not to scratch it. I could see my mom across the room with a glass of wine. But it was never one glass of wine. I was a few years sober then, and I tried not to obsess about her drinking, but I knew where this was going. I ate too much in the hopes that might somehow magically transport me to somewhere where I wasn't pregnant and itchy and watching my mom get obliterated at a wedding in Vermont.

Eventually the toasts came. I grabbed Matt's arm.

He tried to reassure me. "I'm sure it will be fine," he said.

It was not fine. My mother got up and gave a very drunken toast which included the line, "We never thought he'd ever ask her to marry him. It took such a *long* time." She then did a little riff on why he might *not* have wanted to marry her, renumerating my cousin's faults and bad qualities. It was pretty terrible and was the first of many traumatic toasts that Matt had to sit through.

HOW TO LOSE YOUR MOTHER

One of her drunken toasts was such a disaster that she actually (temporarily) got sober afterward. She'd given a toast at a birthday dinner she hosted for her friend Ken Follett. I was not there for that toast because I saw it coming and went into the kitchen to hide. I had gotten really good at avoiding the soul-crushing embarrassment that was the Erica Jong Toast, so whenever I could sense that she was working up to one, I'd wander away. It was one of those toasts in which she got hotter, and angrier, and crazier as she kept going. At some point, she got to the statement "Ken and I never fucked." She was then in her seventies. He was also in his seventies. His wife, a member of Parliament, was there too, and slack-jawed in horror.

After the toast, Matt came into the kitchen, looking ashen.

"Oh, Moll," he said.

"Can we go home now?" I asked.

The following morning, Ken (the other Ken—my stepfather) begged her to stop drinking. He was usually okay with the drunken speeches, and with the drunkenness in general, but this time crossed the line.

And then she was sober—for a while.

About six months after the Follett Fiasco, a cousin hosted Passover dinner. We were all sitting at long tables, listening to someone read the Haggadah. Mom was not drinking. She was still apparently sober. That's what she had been telling everyone.

"I feel so good when I don't drink!" she announced to the table. "I'm so clear!"

"Well, let's go to a meeting then," I replied under my breath. I was at the time maybe twenty years sober, sober long enough to know that trying to get other people sober who didn't want to was a fool's errand.

Of course, she'd always refuse to go. Occasionally, she'd tell me that she loved AA and found it helpful, but mostly I'd get the same old story.

During this Passover dinner, Matt happened to be seated next to Mom. There's a part of the Seder dinner called the Plagues, during which you're supposed to dip your finger (or, better yet, the edge of a knife) into your glass of wine. Each dip represents a Plague. There are ten Plagues, from Frogs to Locusts. Mom started dipping her finger in her red wine glass. I never use wine for the Plagues—just grape juice. But Mom wanted to pretend she was normal, so she had wine. But then she started licking the wine from her finger. It went on and on like this, just dipping and licking. I could see Matt freaking out. Across the table, he looked horrified. And then my mother tipped the glass of wine into her mouth and drank the whole thing in one gulp.

Later, Matt announced, "She's drinking again, Moll."

"No shit," I said.

I asked him if he remembered when we met and I told him that my mom was an alcoholic and he told me I was being silly.

I felt badly for him, I really did. Marrying into an alcoholic family was unbelievably traumatic.

So that was the end of my mom's sobriety.

Between my mother's persistent writing about me, and the constant drunken scenes, I found myself in a perpetual state of worry and embarrassment. Eventually, I just gave up on what the outside world thought of me. Eventually, I adopted this weird coping mechanism in which I just assumed that no one cared about me, and that if they did, they hated me. It was the most negative possible way to read my situation, but it saved me from being a total sociopathic narcissist.

HOW TO LOSE YOUR MOTHER

One of the other ways I survived: I never let myself connect with other people. I mean, it made sense. I had a mother who was completely impenetrable: always drunk, or dreaming, or working, or on a trip. I had a father who, in my heart, I felt had moved on. I had a nanny whom I loved dearly, but who was doing a job for money. (In hindsight, I do think she actually loved me.)

I still have real problems connecting with other humans. Still, even after forty-four years on this planet, I can't really make connections with other people. Sometimes I try, often I don't. I do like people, and sometimes they like me, but deep down there is a wall, a wall that protects me from the danger that is connection. This seems to be true in my relationships with absolutely everyone except my own children. My love for my children is completely bottomless. But for every other person, there's a feeling that they could disappear, could be snatched from this planet, and I would be just fine without them.

I remember growing up thinking I would die if my mom died. But why? Why would that have been true? She barely interacted with me, except to tell me how much she loved me and how much she missed me, which I always found really confusing because if she missed me so much couldn't she just come home? It wasn't like she was in the war or something.

But this baffling emotional dishonesty made me perpetually confused. What was true? What was real? Was my mother's inability to connect with me all in my head? Was this maybe my problem and not hers? After all, people would always tell me how much my mom loved me, because she would tell them how much she loved me. But I never felt very loved.

Does my pathetical inability to connect make me a bad person?

After Matt's CAT scan, I went out to dinner with a friend who works at *The New York Times*.

He happens to have a narcissistic father. He had just called my mom to interview her for a piece he was working on, he asked for her memory of an event, and as they spoke, he realized that she had no recollection whatsoever of this event. But she also seemed to have absolutely no interest in this long-ago story at all, or indeed any curiosity about the piece at all.

After dinner, my friend and I walked up Broadway. I had a question for him.

"How do you know if a narcissist has dementia?"

"It's impossible to tell."

He was, of course, right.

***

I went to the White House Correspondents' Dinner because I need nine guests a week for my podcast. I also went because I actually really love DC. I'm the only person I know who genuinely likes DC; even the people who pretend to love it hate it. Everyone hates DC. Everyone hates "the Swamp." Everyone's favorite things to complain about in DC are, in this order: DC, the people, the "fashion," the swampy corruption of Exxon lobbyists buying dinner for senators, and newsletters funded by chemical companies. It's not necessarily that the corruption in DC is worse than in good old NYC; it's just that it's so very blatant.

Little did I know that, in DC, I would find myself low-key stalked by Kellyanne Conway. A few things about the sunken-eyed mistress of alternative facts. I am friendly with her husband. I think George is a pretty good guy. Was he involved in the

HOW TO LOSE YOUR MOTHER

Federalist Society? Yes! Was he anti-choice? Yes! Was he like all the Never-Trump Republicans? Yes! But I can't help it. I like George. I knew Kellyanne Conway hated me because I was friends with George. But if I had understood the extent of her loathing, I might not even have gone to DC in the first place.

But since I've been doing more political stuff, I've gotten used to being hated. At CPAC, I've been screamed at by far-right-wing writers with crazy eyes. I've gotten scores of death threats. I even had a 4chan thread devoted to killing me. But I've never had a member of Trumpland so obsessed with me. Usually, people are pretty nice to each other in private. Maybe that's just the performative nature of politics.

Kellyanne was at every White House Correspondents' party, behind every corner. Everywhere I went, I would look around and see Kellyanne Conway behind me, glaring. Was she following me? I told people I thought she was following me and everyone said I was crazy. But then, at a predinner reception, she walked up to me and declared, "You're a mess."

Later, when she walked by, she laughed at me.

I was feeling so depleted from Matt's cancer and the huge question mark about his health, everything involving my parents, my mother. A few days before, Mom had called me and threatened to escape from the nursing home. No, I wasn't able to snap back the way I used to. I took the early train home. I ate the blue cheese from the cheese plate, and I hate blue cheese.

I visited my mom and stepdad at the nursing home. Rooms 703 and 705. I brought Bucephalus the Dog and my younger son to distract them, and me. It is easier if I'm not alone with them these days.

Despite the expense of the nursing home it, well, it does have a . . . *smell*—a bad, kind of gross, kind of grim smell. And were those garbage bags of used diapers in the halls?

Ken looked much better. He was watching a musical on TV with his new aide, Johnny.

I sat down.

"I don't want to nag you about when I'm going home," Ken said, "but when am I going home?"

I looked at my son, who was petting the dog. My parents' apartment was going to go on the market soon. It had been cleaned and fixed and painted white. A lot of their stuff was gone, but I still had some crap—books, papers, clothes—to sort through. Everything had been set into motion. There was no way to undo it now.

"Not today," I said. I paused. "But why do you want to move back?"

"Because all my stuff is there," he said.

But there was no stuff waiting for them. Their whitewashed apartment showed almost no trace of the thirty years they'd spent there.

I could feel myself retract. Selling and throwing out their stuff had been a deeply painful and unpleasant experience. But I had still done it as soon as I possibly could. I was the one who had put them into this little hospital. And now that their stuff was gone there was no life to go back to.

I was wearing my mother's opal ring. The Sotheby's guy said it wasn't good enough to sell. I wore it because I felt as if I should get something out of this deal where I took care of the parents who never took care of me. Also, the ring really is beautiful, and looking at it reminds me that I can have at least one nice thing.

HOW TO LOSE YOUR MOTHER

Mom was staring at my finger.

"Did I give that to you?" she asked.

I slid the ring off my finger and into my pocket. I did a quick change of the subject. She had not given me the ring. She had not given me anything. I was supposed to be *watching* her things. *Watching* her ring. But I had *taken* it. None of this was mine.

9

"Well, I won't be getting any bad news until tomorrow," Matt said as he left for a blood draw.

My eyes were, as always, welling up with tears. We live in Metastatic World now. Metastatic World involves a lot of scans. These scans will reveal if the treatment is working or if it's time to "take that big trip" and "get our affairs in order." Of course, Matt has a very slow-moving cancer, so it wouldn't ever be that dramatic; we'd likely have years of various things not working before he dies, but that doesn't make these scans any less horrible.

That night is a Monday night. I go to sleep because I can't stand being awake anymore. I have started doing this, just going to sleep because I can't possibly bear any more consciousness. I don't go to sleep because I'm tired, or even because I particularly want to go to sleep, but instead because I just don't want to be awake. Something has happened to me. I suspect that I am very depressed, but Susan C. suggests I'm in some kind of shock. I can't eat. Like I literally can't eat. People keep asking me if I'm on Ozempic, but I'm not. I'm on the grief diet. I'm on the Surrounded by Death Diet, also known as the Everyone Will Be Dead Soon Diet.

But I'm still about ten pounds heavier than when I was on

drugs. Unsurprisingly, I have, or had, an eating disorder. When I was in the process of getting kicked out of Dalton for being dyslexic, Margaret used to bring me these plain bagels, lightly toasted and just dripping with butter. The butter was so salty and so profoundly soothing.

When I was fifteen, my mom's diet doc gave me diet pills. I loved them. They made me feel great. I became addicted to them. Then when I was sixteen, I became addicted to exercise. I was an exercise-bulimic. Exercise-bulimia is the best kind of bulimia because it seems as if you're really doing something, but what you're doing is nothing: overeating / working out, overeating / working out, repeat this cycle ad infinitum. For years I was one of those fat girls who punished herself in the gym. Hours on the treadmill, then cake. Hours on the stationary bike, then ice cream. Hours of suffering, then minutes of pleasure, but never thin, just very, very tired. Even into my adulthood, I continued in this strange miserable dance with food and exercise. I was healthy because I worked out for hours a day. I destroyed running shoes. But there was part of me that felt entitled, that feel like I could destroy myself with food later.

Then one day I stopped exercising and my life changed. My shrink told me for years to stop exercising, but I was sure that exercise was the thing that kept me from being fat. What I didn't realize was that exercise was actually the thing that kept me from being thin. A strange paradox. Now I don't exercise. I should no longer fear eating, but I just don't feel like eating now.

I drink coffee. I have lattes and iced tea and lemonade. I have ice cream for dinner, but I no longer believe that food will stop the pain. There is a pain in me. Pain like a low ache, like a sunburn or something but it comes from inside. It hurts, it feels like part of me is rotting or sick. Thinking about my mother hurts. I try to remember if thinking about my mother always hurt or if this pain is new and exquisite in its newness. Am I suffering more than I did when I was young?

Maybe?

There was some good news: we wouldn't have to travel for July Fourth weekend—which somehow is a week, July Fourth *week*—because Matt would be busy getting the cancer in his liver nuked. It will be the summer of Sloan Kettering! I've always hated traveling for the Fourth of July anyway.

I went back to my longtime shrink, Dr. Bower. He asked how I was.

"I'm okay," I said. I was weeping.

"You can't possibly be okay," he said.

On a Monday in June, I experienced one of those sleeps so characteristic of Metastatic World. My dreams were similar in spirit and tone to the other truly terrible time in my life: my childhood. I dreamed that I was in the childhood home again, the one on Davis Hill Road, in Connecticut. The one I hated so much. The one at which the stalker Bates used to sit in the driveway. I was scared. I was always scared in that house. And of course my certainty that I'd be murdered by Charles Manson didn't help, either.

At 7:45 a.m. we were at Sloan Kettering. Why different parts of Sloan Kettering occupy different parts of Manhattan, and different styles of buildings, is something never explained to me. The Irish doctor was delighted.

"You read it on the portal!" she said.

We didn't. There is an internet portal on which you can see results, but often these results are written in a terrifying way, filled with doctor-speak that make you positive the patient is going to die within seconds.

"We're too scared to read the portal," Matt said.

"*Well*," the doctor replied, "the lanreotide is working."

This is a big deal. A lot has been riding on this drug working and it is, apparently, working.

"We can talk about using a bland embolization on the met in the liver," she continued.

"A bland embolization": the words delight Matt because they are so filled with meaning and so poetic. I'm reminded all over again why I love him. He has one of those amazing brains. A lot of the time being married to the smartest person I know isn't all that fun, but then other times you remember: he is a person unlike anyone else, he is someone astounding, someone whose DNA is slightly magic. All these years of my mother telling me, based on zero evidence, that I was brilliant, but I had married someone who actually *was* brilliant. Matt has always occupied a completely different intellectual plane.

The problem was I needed him to continue on this one.

So many years of shared history with Matt. There in the doctor's office, I found myself thinking about the first time Matt met my grandpa Howard.

At the end of his life, Grandpa lived in an unremarkable two-story home in Old Greenwich, Connecticut. Dad would take me to visit him. It was one of those houses that was fundamentally wrong, designed wrong and built on the wrong spot—the living room was on the top floor, which was also the first floor, and there were bedrooms on the bottom floor, which was aboveground because the house was built into a hill. It occurs to me that one of the very weird things about the homes of my childhood was that many of them were just slightly off, slightly unlivable, slightly undoable. My grandfather's house comes to me sometimes in dreams, the ugly strangeness of it.

But this wrongness fits, because everything about this chapter is wrong. Grandma had died of cancer when she was only in her early seventies. She was the person who made Grandpa bearable. She was the person other people liked. Was she also the love of Raymond Carver's life? Maybe. That was the story anyway. As always with my family, there were so many lies that it was impossible to know what really ever happened, and, honestly, conjecture is probably more interesting than the truth.

But many of the facts of Grandpa's life *were* legitimately fascinating. He was a dedicated Communist with an FBI file. He spent three months in prison in 1950 for pleading the Fifth before the House Un-American Activities Committee, those cronies of Senator Joseph McCarthy. He had an affair with a woman who would go on to marry Alger Hiss.

I'm trying to remember when I realized my grandpa was famous, or had been famous at one time. There were certainly clues. In his house were posters of movies he'd written or that had been based on his books. There was the Emmy, a brass object that sat on a shelf in the living room. There were other prizes on the shelf behind the piano, and then the ironically named Stalin Peace Prize, which sat on the piano. And then there were the documentary crews. Grandpa always seemed to be talking to some group of shabby-looking people—men with creative facial hair who wanted to know what it was like being part of history. The problem for Grandpa, and for the rest of us, is that history is in the past.

Grandpa was very interesting to people who didn't know

him. His stories were parts of history, things you'd read in books. But to people who knew—his children, his grandchildren, his few remaining friends—he was a tremendous bore. He had an almost pathetic need to keep you hostage—a captive audience for his tales.

On what turned out to be one of the last times I saw Grandpa, I brought Matt to meet him. Matt was excited to meet the great Howard Fast.

"Hello, Matty boy," the great Howard Fast said. He had that kind of very leathery skin and that male-pattern baldness that many Jewish men have. He lit a cigarette. Matt immediately started coughing. At that time, Matt had lost only one aunt and one uncle of cancer. He would eventually lose the rest of them. "What happened to Ryan?" Grandpa asked, checking out Matt from head to toe.

Ryan was an ex-boyfriend, and he had been a literary agent. Matt was an academic, but literary agent was much more useful for Grandpa.

"We broke up, Grandpa," I said.

"Why?" he asked, taking another long drag of his cigarette.

Did he actually even care why Ryan and I broke up? I told him we just kind of got bored with each other. Isn't that generally why people break up?

"What do *you* do?" he asked Matt. "Are you a literary agent?"

"He's not a literary agent, Grandpa."

"*Oh.*"

"But I *am* a fan," Matt smartly said, saving this whole exchange.

Grandpa glowed.

"Tell me. What's your favorite book of mine?"

Grandpa was nothing if not predictable.

Dad and I left Matt with him. We'd heard all his stories before and knew everything he would say. Our interest in hearing these stories for the thousandth time was not enormous.

My father and I sometimes bond over the fact that we're two children of powerful same-sex parents. Part of our shared makeup is that we're so damaged by those same-sex parents that we don't fight back much. We don't have the drive, the rage, the fury to retaliate. We prefer to hide instead. I'm not saying that my mother was ever as bad or as crushing as my grandfather was to my father. It's just that Dad and I have always known that we can't win against these people.

Grandpa died not long after that, when I was pregnant. Soon all my grandparents would be dead. The thing about having living grandparents means that you're young. Having living grandparents means you're not going to be the next to die. Having living grandparents means you've got decades and decades left on this planet, it means your skin is still dewy. Having living grandparents means you are still young. Mine are all dead because I am no longer young. And just like my mother and my grandfather, the two who couldn't get over not being famous, I can't get over not being young. I thought I would be young forever. Time betrayed me. Just as it betrayed everyone else.

My mother's apartment languished on the market, as apartments old people lived in tend to do. I've been spending a lot of time trying to remember the apartment when we moved into it, after the Chucky candy bar people moved out. I'm trying to remember the little family we tried to be. Every week, Sherry-Lehmann delivered a case of wine, sometimes two. I remember the boxes outside our front door. What else? My mom always had a dog, but she wasn't really a dog person. I never saw her walk her dogs. Those dogs were like me: objects, accessories to add color and relatability to an otherwise work-centered life.

This is not a criticism of a work-centered life; I live one, too. It is 7:55 p.m. on a summer Friday and I've been up since 4:50 a.m., working. I am not at a party. I am not rowing in a lake with a kid. I am not at a dinner. I am not cooking hot dogs on a fire in the Catskills. I am working. But I like to think of myself as someone who would walk that dog.

What was it like to be young in the white brick building at 150 East Sixty-Ninth Street, on the twenty-seventh floor? I'm trying to remember who that girl is, or was. The main thing I remember about my teenage years was my struggle with obsessive-compulsive disorder. I was so obsessive, so worried about everything. Some of the ways the compulsive disorder manifested was with checking, checking in closets and under beds and in drawers. Was the stove off? Was the door locked? Should I check one more time? I should check one more time. Did I leave that cigarette burning in the ashtray?

I was born to privilege, born on third base, but desperate to strike out and go home.

That apartment, which I lived in from the age of twelve until about twenty, that apartment was now staged to look as if a fashionable family lived there. (We'd stashed my parents' own stuff into a couple of rooms.) It was now filled with furniture meant to pantomime the normal life of normal people, the kind of people we never were, and, frankly, never wanted to be.

*

Matt and I set in motion more surgery, more hospital stays, more embolization. But this was good news, this was the best-case scenario. We finally had good news to tell the children.

The chaos of death surrounded me and made it hard to focus, to make choices, stupid choices. Did I get that text message, or did I imagine it? Did I even care? Maybe I didn't. So, I go to sleep. Since I was sleeping too much, I got up during the night, but who cared? I don't know. I used to care about getting up in the middle of the night but not now.

On Wednesday, the city filled with smoke from the wildfires in Canada. The sky turned orange. My asthmatic son couldn't breathe. I walked through the city as if I didn't care because I somehow could no longer connect with my own mortality. Everything seemed impossibly irrelevant. I was unable to connect with the normal stuff of life: crossing the street, answering a call, everything mundane felt oddly inaccessible.

Susan C. and I talked on the phone. She told me that the best writing about nepotism was by Saul Bellow's son Adam. In the late nineties, he wrote an essay for Tina Brown for her long-departed magazine *Talk*. Susan warned me that the piece wasn't online.

I did something I didn't want to do: I sent Adam Bellow a LinkedIn message. I hate LinkedIn, absolutely despise it—an entire world of people who work for companies and went to college—two things I completely don't relate to. Adam replied and kindly sent me a PDF of the piece about his father, which included the best paragraph about growing up with a writer-parent that I've ever read:

> It may be difficult for someone who hasn't grown
> up with a writer in the family to conceive the many

ways in which a novel can become part of your life. There is the discipline of writing, to begin with, and the procreative hush that it imposes on the literary household. There is also the reception of the book, which in my father's case was almost always a major event. But for those who were involved in its creation, a great novel can take on a life of its own. For them it becomes like a flesh-and-blood person, a character in their lives, a dubious addition to the family. Such is my relationship to *Herzog*.

I invited Adam Bellow to meet me for a drink at my old-man club in Midtown. We sat at a big table in the room with the fireplace. We chatted. He had the confidence of someone who had been handsome in his youth. I never had that confidence. I find those who have it jarring and a little weird. He was maybe in his sixties now. He kept taking his glasses on and off.

At some point, the conversation with Adam took a wrong turn, and I started talking about my parents, and my husband, and all my tragedy porn. I could feel myself welling up. I had gotten increasingly amazing at swallowing tears. I could swallow all the tears. I could make them go away.

Adam tried to be soothing, but I'm always suspicious of other nepo babies. He was not totally unthreatening, but not threatening either.

"Are you in therapy?" he asked me.

"I just went back," I said.

"You might be having a midlife crisis," he added.

Was I in the middle of my life? I thought about my life, thought about the years that stretched behind me. The years I'd spent dealing with my mother's drinking, and then the years I spent doing my own drinking, and doing my own disfunction. Did I only have half my life left? How old would I live to be? Would I actually even make it to eighty-eight? Had I wasted my youth? I had been young for so long, and I had missed it. I had forgotten to pay attention. Like all young people, I had thought I would always be young, and now I wasn't young anymore.

I ignored Adam's comment and went off to a dinner I was late for. And then I rudely proceeded to spend most of that dinner on my phone. It wasn't a successful dinner. I wandered off and into a taxi. But hours later, as I sat weeping in the bathtub, I wondered if perhaps I *was* in fact having a midlife crisis.

Sometimes, out of nowhere, I get crushingly depressed. How it comes on is usually some inability to outrun it. The previous night, I'd come home and tried to eat ice cream for dinner, but was too depressed even to eat ice cream, and I threw it out. Then I decided to go to bed because then I didn't have to be awake anymore. In bed, I wept softly so no one could hear. The game is to hide the pain from the teenage occupants of the house. Then I started fantasizing about killing myself. I would jump out the window, I decided, because it's so *Alice in Wonderland*. Something about it is so scary, so terrible, so tragic. Being in AA, you know a lot of people who've killed themselves—usually on pills, but sometimes they've hung themselves, which seems like a lot of work. There's a lot of preparation and planning involved with that method.

On Sunday, I came home from another trip to Washington and the aide texted me: "You have to call your mother. She refuses to bathe. She smells."

HOW TO LOSE YOUR MOTHER

I called the little nursing home apartment. Mom picked up the phone. "Hi, darling," she said in a voice like Daisy Buchanan. Ringing of money and reminding me of my grandfather's dream to breed daughters who didn't seem as if they'd come out of the shtetl, as he had.

Mom has always sounded rich and European. Two things she is not. For a minute, I was again transported to my childhood. For a slip of a second, I was sitting in a five-star hotel with my gorgeous mother. She was wearing gorgeous designer clothing. She was pretending. She was always pretending. But on that day, I almost believed it. I almost believed I was her entire life.

The eighties. My mother always smelled so opulent and extravagant—rare Parisian perfume, before everyone started wearing Opium and Chanel No. 5. Growing up, I wondered how such a glamorous person had birthed me.

For a moment on the phone, she wasn't a demented shell of herself, but was instead a glamorous ingénue hanging out with movie stars and judging film festivals. For a minute, the lie of the great Erica Jong was back.

But then she started talking and it was clear she had no idea where she was.

Matt's dad had been hovering between life and death for three months in an unremarkable hospital in Bridgeport, Connecticut. Matt says that the doctors have wanted to take out the tube and give his father too much morphine, but Matt refuses. "I will not euthanize my dad," he says.

We had euthanized one of our dogs in the fall of 2022. My younger son held Cerberus as the life flooded out of him. That line between life and death once crossed never uncrossed. After the deed was done, the lifeless body of Cerberus lay on a table in a room in the animal hospital on the FDR Drive. My son and I were crying so hard we couldn't see. Matt had tears streaming down his cheeks. What we didn't know was that it would be a year of death, of surgeries, of hospitalizations, of waiting in doctors' offices. We didn't know that Cerberus was a harbinger. But that's the thing about harbingers: you never know until it's too late.

Cerberus now lives where the dead pets do, wherever that is. With my dead grandparents, and my friends who died of drug overdoses, and my sponsee who drank herself to death. All these dead are somewhere. Or maybe they're nowhere.

Actually, I think Cerberus's ashes are on the shelf next to my grandfather's Emmy. But the ashes are just ashes.

I think a lot about death. Sitting in the waiting room, looking at all the people who are twenty, thirty years older than Matt. They just want a little more time, but then again we all just want a little more time. In their fancy nursing home, all my mom and stepfather *have* is time. Days are spent trying to find creative ways to run out the clock, to keep the patients busy as they descend into those last few months or years. Mom and Ken read the paper. They watch cable news. They fritter the time away.

I think a lot about how little time any of us have left.

Did Covid kill my mom and stepfather? Technically no, functionally yes. I remember a phone call we had right before the interminable lockdowns.

"I'm going to dinner with some friends from Milan," she'd said.

"No, Mom. Please don't. There is this terrible virus coming from Milan, coming from Italy. It's killing people. Please, Mom, don't go to that dinner. You need to be careful. It's killing older people."

Those first few months of Covid were a wash of obituaries and dead fathers. Those first few months of Covid were marked by empty streets and kids lying on the sofa watching television. At first it was scary, thinking we were all going to die. Then it was cozy, not needing to be anywhere. So much of American life was about needing to be somewhere, and then all of a sudden, we didn't need to be anywhere. Then it was boring. Then it was scary. Then it was the end of my parents.

They became too good at quarantining. They just stayed home forever and ever. They drank, and watched TV, and stopped pretending that they could exist in society. They slept until noon and slid into their illnesses. They never came back from quarantine. They never came out of it.

I knew some people who died of Covid, mostly fathers. But the more subtle losses, like the loss of my parents, those are harder to quantify. They blur into some kind of tapestry of missing pieces, a life that is oddly unconnected to itself.

In January, they found the mass on my husband's pancreas. That same month, we put my mother and stepfather in a nursing home. By "we," I mean "me." It's me, always me; there is no we. I am an only child. I am the only bit of Erica Jong in the universe except for her, but she sits in a nursing home on Second Avenue reading and rereading the newspaper.

I knew there was no way that grief would come for me, too. I had spent my entire life trying to get away from the loneliness of being abandoned by my parents. I assumed this would somehow preclude me from mourning their deaths. Like with almost everything in my life, I was deeply wrong. You can't pre-grieve your parents much as you might want to, or need to. As an addict, I was always looking for a quick fix, a way to skip the hard work. I was the second or third generation in the family to love diet pills. I would take them instead of eating. You can cheat your weight, but you can't cheat grief. Even if your parents never loved you, or you never loved them, or some weird combination of the two, grief still comes for all of us.

I was at Sloan Kettering, sitting in an elegantly modern waiting room with a view of the East River. I was looking at my phone, waiting for Matt to have the met in his liver blandly embolized with little bits of glass. Imagine paying someone to shoot glass into the cancer in your liver. The cancer, the one-centimeter tumor, is called a met and it is either *in* his liver or *on* his liver depending whom you ask. I don't know how to spell it. Is it met, mette, mett? It stands for metastasis.

It was mid-July, and most of polite society had left the hot concrete for their summer adventures. I was writing my *Vanity Fair* column from the modern Sloan Kettering waiting room. Fancy people get cancer and they donate gobs of money to hospitals and doctors in the hopes that this will allow them to cheat death, but just like grief, death still comes for all of us, too.

Then. A week later, another very hot July day. I had been trying not to go to parties while my father-in-law was lying in a coma, but he'd been in and out of this coma for months, and my not-going-to-parties resolve had faded. So of course I was at a party, a book party, when it happened. It was at the home of a billionaire, and the book was about Bitcoin. The author was also an actor, and he gave a very long speech about how great he was for wanting to write a book. I was of course thinking about this book you are now, for better or worse, reading. This book was now going to destroy my life, I had decided. This book about the myriad ways I had betrayed my mother, and the strategies I had used to stay alive. I had a little bit of survivor's guilt about my childhood, I guess. How had *I* been the one to make it out alive, and my own mother, who was during my childhood, bigger and stronger and smarter and famous, sitting in a nursing home picking the skin off her scalp? How had I survived my childhood, and she had not? When she was the one who had created my childhood?

Anyway, it was a pretty good party; I had a nice time.

But then I got a text from Matt:

"My father died."

I had actually started to believe that he might not ever die, that he might get better, or maybe would just hang out forever in that suspended state. Despite everything, his death was still slightly shocking.

Stu had been my father-in-law for twenty years and then he was gone. Matt still had cancer, but Stu was dead. He was ninety-one. Ninety-one is too old to be a tragic death, but all death is in its own way tragic and there was still a feeling that he'd been swept off this earth. Just swept off the face of this planet. He'd fallen at home, and then a cascade of different bodily failures followed. The body failed, one organ at a time.

My mother-in-law wept many tears. She was attended by nurses. They made her use a wheelchair so she too wouldn't fall and die. My mother-in-law has now survived all her sisters, her husband, his siblings. She's the last now.

At the funeral, Matt spoke about how much he loved his dad. Our younger son, who was very close with his grandfather, also spoke. While Matt had lost a father, our son had lost a best friend. Growing up, I had been very close with my own grandmother, Bette Fast. I had spent many weeks sleeping in the Fast apartment on Fifth Avenue and Seventy-Ninth Street. I'd always desperately wished that *she* had been my mother—the serene, elegant redheaded sculpture. Imagine having a mother who was capable of mothering. Being in that apartment always felt like a dream. It was an odd thing, growing up in a family that prized fame so highly, and wishing that you were the child of one of the nonfamous members. Grandma Bette died of cancer when I was a freshman in high school. Fourteen years old, a few months younger than our son when his beloved grandfather died.

I did not give a eulogy at my father-in-law's funeral. I felt very badly about this, but I just wasn't up to it. As everyone else spoke, I thought about my mom. At least she wasn't there to give a speech about herself. I also thought about myself, about how if I were a bigger person, I should have been able to deliver a profound, heartfelt eulogy at my father-in-law's funeral. Despite an adulthood engaged in the project of trying to change myself, I was still the same person I'd always been. The person hidden by the cupcakes and phobias; the person who wanted to buy that haunted palazzo and burn it down. I used to joke that if Mom couldn't sell her house in Weston, I would set fire to it. I would wonder if destroying the house would somehow release me. Could I obliterate these artifacts and finally be free?

We buried my father-in-law in the same cemetery where my grandfather Howard Fast was buried. My father-in-law admired Howard Fast so much that he had bought the adjacent cemetery plots. But for some reason no one in my family had ever bought Grandpa a headstone. Grandma Bette had a stone, but Grandpa Howard did not. No, there was nothing, nothing at all, marking the notorious, impossible, once-famous Howard Fast's time on this earth.

10

I was on a Zoom with two very well-intentioned women. It was Mom's sixtieth Barnard reunion. My mom loves Barnard. She has always been very proud that she's an alumna. When she was a student there, she dated the man who would become her first husband, a schizophrenic who tried to push her out of a window on Central Park West to see if she could fly. Years later, Mom would receive a letter that he had died. She didn't weep. She just put the letter down and went about her business.

These Barnard ladies wanted Mom to give a speech at the reunion.

I explained that Mom was not in any universe capable of giving a speech. She has dementia, I explained.

The ladies, however, wouldn't hear of that. This is something I've noted about the way famous people are regarded—non-famous people often can't accept that the rules of human existence still actually apply to famous people. Such is the power of fame: because my mother is, or was, famous, it's almost as if she's post-human.

"Oh, your mom will be fine," one of the ladies said. "The moderator is great."

I pondered this comment: a moderator so great that she

can somehow overcome dementia. Against my better judgment, I acquiesced and accepted the invitation on my mother's behalf. Erica Jong would be the featured speaker at the sixtieth Barnard reunion. She appeared to understand what this event would involve, and seemed excited about the whole thing. It felt important to let her do it. I wanted her to have something to look forward to.

On the day of the reunion, I walked over to the nursing home—it's a few blocks north from my apartment, and a couple blocks east. The lady at the front desk swiped me in, lest I forget my mother and stepfather are in a place they can't leave. I took the elevator upstairs. Mom wasn't dressed. The aide was concerned that she hadn't showered, yet again. In the closet, I located one of my mother's favorite dresses, and handed it to her.

I asked her to get dressed. I reminded her about the reunion, and the speech.

She walked into the other room. There was something so crushing about her current state, something so exquisitely painful about this condition of being both living and dead. She was a zombie . . . but she was also my mom? Sort of.

She came back into the living room, still in her pajamas. Somehow she has gone from Daisy Buchanan to F. Scott Fitzgerald to Zelda in just a few short years.

"I'm nervous," she said.

Even she knew she shouldn't be giving any speeches.

"Don't worry," I said in a soothing voice. "I'll take care of you. I'll make sure to bring you back here." I wasn't as resentful in that moment as I would become later in the evening, when I thought back to all the times I'd wait for her to pick me up from school, and it would turn out to be Margaret. Or just no one.

She seemed comforted by the idea that I'd be there to take care of her.

We got a taxi. She was anxious. She complained about being dizzy. She's always dizzy now. We had nothing to talk about during the ride because I didn't want to have to talk about everything she doesn't remember. I looked out the window and blurred my eyes. I was sad. I'm always sad when I'm with her. It used to be more simple—I used to just be panicked that she would do something embarrassing. Now I don't feel like that anymore. Now I'm just sad about the soul draining from her body.

We arrived at Barnard. When we got out of the taxi, there was someone waiting for us—one of those efficient, pretty people who is always greeting you. She took us to a room. We made chitchat and the room slowly filled with women. They were my mother's age, or younger. Okay, most of them were younger. Some of them may have known her personally, but it was impossible to tell. Mom has always done this thing of pretending she knows everyone. I think it's a famous person thing, because recently people have started coming up to me, and I just pretend I know them. It's better to lie. Otherwise, they will probably be offended. In this way, I'm becoming just like my mother.

When we were setting up her place on the stage, Mom said, "I didn't have many friends in college. Mostly I was with my boyfriend."

How did she remember this? And it was also an impressively self-aware analysis. Of course she always lived her life for men.

I was overcome with anxiety. Would Mom be able to give the speech, or were we going to experience a nuclear meltdown?

She got up onstage. They asked me to sit next to her; I guess the thinking was that I could wrestle the mic from her if things went really off the rails.

As predicted, the moderator was not able to prevent Mom from being demented. But another thing about the power of fame is that audiences just seem to like to watch famous people, no matter what they do. Even though Mom couldn't remember much and her head was full of snakes, she was plausible enough. She spoke in the empty platitudes of a fortune cookie. "You need to be brave!" Mom announced triumphantly. The crowd ate it up. Everyone applauded. Even my cousin, who knows Mom is demented, was impressed. I was both baffled and relieved.

She squeezed out a few more platitudes and then, mercifully, it was over. I sweated through my T-shirt. My mouth was completely dry. If an event can take years off your life, this one definitely did.

But she seemed to love the whole experience. I'd been a good daughter. And I guess that was something.

As we were leaving, the Barnard ladies gave us a T-shirt with a famous quote of my mom's on the front: IF YOU DON'T RISK ANYTHING, YOU RISK EVEN MORE.

We folded ourselves back into a taxi.

"I need a drink," she declared.

I thought to myself: *I need an AA meeting.*

So much of our lives have been about alcohol that it makes me want to cry.

I had started to feel a pull toward Europe. Toward the Adriatic, toward Venice. I love Venice. It's the Disneyland of the Adriatic. Maybe it's wildly out of fashion, but it doesn't matter, for me it is some kind of piece of the puzzle. There is some kind of unfinished business there, some kind of unfinished something that haunts me. Venice is under my skin, in the way places get under your skin when you have one of those unresolved childhoods that you can't stop reliving. Every year, when it starts getting warmer, I again long for the smell of Venetian summer sewage. The streets of Venice smell not that differently from the streets of New York in the summer: sewage that stings the nostrils. It is a strange summer passion, Venice, but I feel stuck in it. My ache for Venice is like some kind of bougie muscle-memory.

I started going to Venice as a child because my mother had a lover there. He was Italian (obviously) and he was married to a rich German woman who was maybe a countess. Did the countess know my mother was having sex with her husband? Perhaps.

The countess was matronly, and my mother was sexy. The countess was rich, and my mother was, well, not rich. The countess was old, and my mother was young . . . well, maybe not young, but at least *younger*.

Perhaps coming to Venice at forty-four was my way of trying to fix my childhood, to unlive those unhappy days. I know that I'm still a little stuck. Maybe the difference between a bad childhood and a good childhood is that you never escape a bad childhood. Years later you're still trying to fix it. Like many people with my condition, a condition I am loath to diagnose but is something between being traumatized and being traumatizing, I keep reliving parts of my childhood in the hopes of fixing them or ironing them out, of winning them.

So I needed to come back to Venice.

A few days before my son and I left, I talked to my dad on the phone. I love my dad, although I do think it was his idea to serve me carrot cake on my first birthday. But there is something, some kind of power my mother had over me that my dad did not. I read Freud when I was growing up. I was told every girl was in love with her father. I was not. I was just overwhelmed by my mother. Is that the same thing as love?

Howard Fast, much like Erica Jong, had been an absolutely crushing human being to have as a parent. My grandpa was very competitive with my dad. He couldn't share. He was always worried that if my dad got famous, he (my grandpa) would become less famous. He was worried Dad would steal his fame, like something out of a Norse myth. There was only one Fast who could occupy the bestseller list and that Fast was Howard. I didn't see it firsthand, but my dad always conveyed the humiliation.

My mom, though impossible, wasn't like that. She loved the idea of my being famous, because I was one of her accessories. My being famous would be just more opportunity for *her* to get more famous. Mom always thought dynastically.

When I was young, I couldn't connect with my dad about all this, but as I've gotten older, this is a subject we bond over. My father and I were, and are, very different people. My dad has a moral core, a kind of spirituality and a quest for joy that I do not have. I'm not even sure I'd want it. Which is perhaps not the greatest self-analysis.

"I put Mom in a home, and I don't feel that bad," I told my father. "I actually feel kind of great." I was walking down the street, wondering if anyone was listening to my end of the conversation. If anyone did, I'm sure they thought I was a very terrible person, the most terrible person in the world.

I wanted my dad to know that I felt guilty and that I understood it was no coincidence that the moment I moved Mom into a home, I started to spiral into the worst depression of my life.

But that depression was also punctuated by the most amazing feeling, a feeling which can best be described as relief: I had survived them, my mother and Ken.

"When your grandfather died," my dad said, "I had the same feeling."

Which was?

"The feeling that only one of us is going to get out alive. And I want it to be me."

It's funny having a father who went through exactly the same experience with his own father. It's not the usual nepotism; it's more like a kind of death match. You know there isn't room on this planet for both of you. For a long time, my mother had always been the winner, and then one day, things changed.

In late July, Matt's cancer was getting better. The treatment was working, and he was slowly coming back to being himself. He was still fragile, but not as fragile as he had once been. He would be okay without me for several days. Wouldn't he?

I tried to schedule the Venice trip during what should have been one of the quietest weeks of the summer. Also, it was a nonelection year, which also should have meant less drama. But of course I landed in Venice to a superseding indictment, and a few days later came Trump's second federal indictment, and the way more serious counts of interfering with the certification of the 2020 election.

My son and I went together. It was just a few days after my father-in-law died, so the timing was not exactly the greatest. Did this trip make any sense at all? Leaving Matt and his cancer, right after his father died? It felt cruel. It felt like something my mom might do. I've never entirely known how to be human, not really, but at least I knew that if any behavior or activity seemed like something my mother would do, I should probably do the opposite.

But the reservation was nonrefundable, and, as I kept reminding myself, I had had an epically bad year—a no-good, very bad year, if you will—not of course as bad as Matt's year, but really quite hideously bad. You know, the kind of year people write memoirs about. In other words, I was burned out.

People were constantly telling me that I needed a vacation (when, that is, they weren't telling me I needed to go back to therapy). During those months between Matt's diagnosis and my father-in-law's death, during those months, people would always ask me how I was. On the rare occasion when I would tell them the truth, they would usually respond with some variation on "Perhaps you'd want to find someone to talk to about this? Maybe you should be in therapy?"

So, against my better judgment, to Venice I went.

I am "in recovery" from my fear of flying. I was grounded for one entire decade, too scared to fly. It was terrible. During those years I couldn't fly, everything felt small, rickety, dangerous. Bridges were death traps. Trains were projectiles of terror. Boats and cars were doom-buggies. Life got smaller and smaller. Life felt as if it were happening inside a postage stamp. I was afraid of things I had never thought to be afraid of. When I finally forced myself to start flying again, it was a revelation. No, that's not big enough—it was a religious experience.

Now I still obsess, but I can actually go places. The worst part, though, about being too scared to fly is that the fear doesn't ever go away. Instead, it gets worse, it slides into other things, like driving a car, riding in boats, crossing bridges, being alone. I always thought that I could isolate the fear of flying and stop feeling it, but that's not how it works. The fear has just grown and grown and there is no way to solve the fear but to go through it. This is what I've learned with exposure therapy. As with so many things (like getting sober), feeling feelings is the only way. Unfortunately for me, and for everyone else, the only way through is through. I am still scared of flying, but I now know the only way through is through.

Obviously, given that my mom wrote *Fear of Flying*, this is all feels a little too on-the-nose. She wrote *Fear of Flying*, and bequeathed her fear of flying to me, but she was always, always, *always* on an airplane. This was all very confusing. As her accessory, I was often on the same plane, though usually in coach with Margaret while my mother sat in first class.

My son and I arrived in Venice midday, and the sky was clear and blue, and the water smelled cheerfully of sewage. We did the things people do on vacation. We ate lots of meals. We bought clothes. We saw art. We tried to be normal. It was an exercise we did a lot this year, trying to be normal, trying to forget about the cancer growing in his father, trying to forget about his dead grandfather, trying to forget about his grandparents in the nursing home. Trying to be normal, despite all evidence to the contrary.

Italy was always a special place for my mom, and she always considered our trips there bonding time. When I was thirteen, she and I went to Florence and stayed at the medieval villa where she had lived when, as a student at Barnard, she'd studied in Florence. The villa was situated in the hills outside of Florence and had been a private home when she lived there in the sixties, but had long since been turned into a hotel called Torre di Bellosguardo. The hotel didn't have air-conditioning. It was hot. Because I was thirteen, I was cranky and annoying about the whole thing. I was mean to my mom the way teenagers can be. I told her she sucked. I told her I hated her and that she was a bad mother. But she was actually, during that trip, a great mother—all she wanted to do was sit by the pool of the villa she had lived in when she was twenty and tell me wonderful stories about Italy when she was young. She was nice, and loving, on that trip. A normal mom. But at some point she did get so mad at me that she dumped a bottle of Pellegrino on my head. We still laugh about it.

There were many other trips to Italy. When I was a kid, my mom would rent a house near her lover-of-the-moment, near the house his countess-wife bought him to live in. It was a very old crumbling house with air-conditioning in only one room. It was very dusty, and I would sleep in a wobbly old bed that was also insanely dusty. There were rats in my room. (This is in itself not an extraordinary statement. The entire city of Venice is completely filled with rats.)

But my room had wall-to-wall carpeting, and the rats ran through the carpet; they made *tunnels* in the carpet. At night, I would lie in bed and listen to the rats scuffling about. I could hear their little feet on the stone as they slid through the tunnels they'd created in the space between the wall-to-wall carpet and the stone floor. I'd want to get out of bed, but I wouldn't because I was scared of the rats.

Some of the worst experiences of my entire life were in Italy, come to think of it.

I was about fourteen and we were staying at a house in Tuscany. It was owned by friends of my mom's. The man had been a studio executive in the seventies and eighties. I knew something was off when, at dinner, in front of my mother and his wife, he stroked my face and told me how beautiful I was. Maybe my mother and his wife were too drunk to notice. Maybe they noticed and didn't care.

But I wasn't beautiful. I was fat and had acne. He wasn't telling me I was beautiful because he actually thought I was beautiful. He was doing some kind of weird psychological thing with me and his wife and my mother. I didn't know what it was, but I absolutely knew it was wrong, and dangerous, and the kind of thing a parent should protect you from.

Later, I took Mom aside.

"You have to make him stop doing that," I said. "It's so embarrassing."

But Mom was very, very drunk.

"You are beautiful, though," my mom said. "You just don't know it. You are *so* beautiful."

She was slurring. I wasn't beautiful but I didn't care. I didn't need to be beautiful. I was cunning. I could fend for myself. Beauty wasn't that important to me because I'd never had it.

"You need to tell him to stop," I said.

"And *you* need to loosen up."

He tormented me all weekend long. He was waiting for me in the guesthouse. He was waiting for me around the corner, with his enormous hands on my face, telling me I was beautiful. I was a child. I was fourteen.

He didn't rape me. He didn't sexually assault me. But he made me feel deeply unsafe. This experience made me realize that my mother would never protect me and that I had to protect myself. Was that the moment that hardened my heart, made it rocklike? I don't know. I don't think it was one moment in particular; it was a combination of moments that made me so removed, so detached, so alone.

HOW TO LOSE YOUR MOTHER

My son and I left Venice a day early. We went to London. I made an excuse that I had to do some TV interviews in the UK, but that wasn't the truth. I told this lie to my son and to my travel agent. I left because one day I woke up and it felt as if I were being choked by my childhood. Strange: one day I was fine and the next day I couldn't breathe. For the last several years, I'd been going back to Venice and reliving my childhood, but suddenly, after the gentle smell of sewage started to seem inexorable, I understood that I had become like one of those military reenactors. But the war was growing up.

So that last morning, when I woke up, I realized, just like the sour British general, that I wasn't going to win. America was gone just like the seventies were gone—and the eighties, and the nineties, too. The war was over, and I'd lost. And even worse than that, I was stuck shadowboxing a mom who was sitting in a nursing home, staring at a shelf of books she didn't know she wrote.

There was another part of me, a part of me who *was* actually brave, perhaps a destroyer of worlds, a person who realized forward was the only way. That person knew the past was over, that I couldn't try and make peace, I just needed to move on.

A good childhood you want to get back to. But because a bad childhood never ends, I was still tracking down almost-stepdads and making dates with almost-stepsisters. I was always trying to find a way to make peace with the past. But that morning in Venice, I finally realized I had lost. There would be no peace.

And I hadn't even been trying to slay those demons. I was inviting those demons to brunch and buying them little presents.

11

A few days after I returned from Venice, my stepfather's sister—my aunt—died. She was seventy-seven. Old enough not to be tragic, but young enough to still be just a little tragic. They found her on the floor. I wrote her obituary, which turns out to be a task you can't say no to. (Then right after I wrote a column about George Santos. Which project was worse?) My cousin sent me the information for the funeral. The same funeral home my family had used for my father-in-law. I remember reading something about how more people die in the winter, but this summer had already seen the deaths of two of my AA friends (one from a brain tumor and one from drinking themself to death), my father-in-law, and now my aunt.

Not that I wanted to, but I felt I had to go over to the nursing home and see how Ken was coping with his sister's death. I took off my mother's opal ring, which I was now constantly wearing, although it belonged to her. I felt guilty enough to tuck it into my jewelry box before I left. (And no, I still didn't know how to open the safe I had installed in my apartment for my mother's jewelry.)

I walked over to Inspir. I signed in, got a fob, and swiped myself into the elevator. I pressed "7." I swiped into the hall, which was filled with formerly fancy people who now couldn't remember their middle names.

I sat in my parents' little living room. Both of them were there, staring at me.

"How *are* you?" I asked Ken. "I'm sorry about Patty."

"You know, people die," my mom declared.

So she did understand that Patty was no longer with us. And this was classic Mom—although she wasn't really there anymore, the need to make grand pronouncements definitely still was.

"I have to go to the bathroom," she announced suddenly and left the room.

Ken and I had a moment alone.

"You're the healthiest of the siblings now," I told him.

I couldn't believe how uncomfortable I was.

Ken nodded.

"I need a tie for the funeral," he declared. "A *red* tie. That's why you need to move us back to the apartment. All my stuff is there."

I was about to sign a contract on the apartment. I had sold the family home. The ultimate betrayal.

The aide lingered in the hallway. How long would I need to stay before I could consider this visit done? I loved my mom, used to be obsessed with her, I would have given anything in the world to have gotten some time alone with her. As a little girl, I used to sit outside her office, hoping she'd come out and spend time with me. I would fight with Ken for the chance to take a trip alone with her. All I ever wanted was to get her attention and now, all these years later, I didn't want it. I didn't even want to see her. I had missed the party. And now the party was coming to an end.

My mom didn't wish me a happy forty-fifth birthday. She didn't know it was my birthday. I called her, waiting to see if she would say anything about my birthday, but she did not. It was not even clear if she knew who I was.

She is both alive and dead. She is both my mom and not my mom.

We are through, we are over. The mother I was desperate for, that mother, she is gone, and she will never be. We will never have the relationship I desperately wanted. I will never be able to go back and fix it.

My birthday is at the end of the summer, and for years my birthday was celebrated in Italy, with adults. One year, my mother's boyfriend's countess-wife gave me a tin of hard candy. Another year in Italy, another friend of hers gave me a bocci ball set. Must have weighed a hundred pounds. We left the balls behind in the house we were staying in.

I never had a birthday party with people my own age until I was an adult, but I should also point out that I really didn't have a lot of friends. I never related to people my own age: they seemed scary, they knew things, they knew how to be cool. I didn't know how to be cool. I barely knew how to be human.

Until I got sober, I always thought I'd die young. But as I stayed sober, I kept having birthdays. Birthday after birthday. Time continued to march on.

I don't know when it was that I accidentally told someone my mom was dead, or when I started referring to her in the past tense, but at some point, after moving her into Inspir, I started to think of her as dead. I would still visit, and during the visits, I would remind myself, "She is actually not dead." It was around this time that I became convinced I was losing my mind. I started seeing a memory doctor, somebody my mom had refused to see. I started doing little block pattern exercises. I started trying desperately to keep the parts of my brain working, even the parts that did things I didn't really do in adulthood, like block patterns.

I would still sometimes force the children to go visit her and my stepfather on the seventh floor of the nursing home on Second Avenue. They'd lived in the nursing home since January. Ken's Parkinson's was galloping toward its conclusion. Meanwhile my mom mostly watched news and drank coffee and refused to participate in any of the planned activities.

I called her.

"Hi, Mom," I said.

"Hi, darling."

"How are you?"

"When will you come see me?"

"Soon." I was lying. "Very soon. What are you doing now, Mom?"

"I'm just lying down."

"Go back to sleep then."

I will do anything to get her off the phone. I am a bad daughter. I am drowning in the knowledge that I am a bad daughter.

She'd become an airhead, a ditz. When I'd see her in the nursing home, she'd tell me how pretty I was, and how much she liked my jewelry (some of which was her jewelry), and then I would leave, I would wander off back to my apartment.

The tragedy: now I could get her attention, but of course now I didn't want it. My whole relationship with her was like having an inoperable tumor—the dull ache of a love that never was.

I called her to try to tell her that Ken was really sick.

"Mom," I said, "Ken is not forever."

"He's back from the hospital. I've missed him so much. I've missed you, too. My darling."

"Ken is not forever," I repeated.

"I've missed you! I'm *so* glad you're here."

But I wasn't "there"; I was "here," at home.

"Mom, you know what I'm trying to say, right?"

Silence on the line.

"Ken is dying," I said. "He is going to die."

I paused. She paused.

"He is?" she asked.

***

As my son and I went down the hall to my parents' apartment in the nursing home, I noticed that the plaque on the room of Martha Updike, John's widow, was gone. I wondered where Martha Updike was now. She and my mother had been friends, sort of. I made a mental note to ask my mom what she knew about Martha's departure. And then I realized that of course Martha had died.

"We should go to Israel," my mother said when we entered their apartment. CNN was blasting on the TV. Hamas terrorists had just attacked Israel—murdering thousands of people and kidnapping more than two hundred—children, Americans, the elderly. There were videos of a demented granny holding a machine gun. She'd been kidnapped. She was Israeli. She was like my mother: alive but dead. Her granddaughter cried on television, begged for her to be saved, but I wondered, who would she be saving?

"We should be fighting," my mother said.

HOW TO LOSE YOUR MOTHER

It was a Sunday and I'd dragged myself to visit my mom, but first I took off her beautiful ring of green opal. I will admit that I'd come to dread the weekends because the weekends meant I had to visit the mother in her costly modern prison. I'd had a rule: once a week. This had now slid into once every two weeks.

She was a terrible mother, ergo I shouldn't *have* to be a good daughter. But of course I was wracked by guilt. I wasn't a good daughter; she wasn't a good mother, but we were not even. We would never be even. There was no way to get even. That hole in my heart would never be filled no matter how much ice cream and Prada shoes I tried to fill it with. I would always be empty and alone. I would always be a bad daughter.

My mom was wearing the T-shirt the Barnard people had given her, the one with her famous platitude: IF YOU DON'T RISK ANYTHING, YOU RISK EVEN MORE. Mom's hair was unwashed and it clung to her face. She wasn't wearing a bra.

That Israeli grandmother in the hostage video, she was like my mother: no longer in there. I guess I was a bad person for thinking that, a bad daughter for wondering why a demented person at the end of their life was worth the same value as a child at the beginning of theirs. I needed to stop all this obsessing about aging, and death, needed to stop asking the question, "What even is the point of life?" I needed to stop thinking about this as my year of death.

"We should be in Israel," Mom declared to the television.

"Why?" I asked.

"Because we're *Jews*."

I was so delighted that Mom didn't have Twitter anymore. I considered the joys of her weighing in on the nuances of the Israel-Palestine conflict. I thought about her tweeting "Molly and

I are getting on a plane to Israel and we're joining the IDF." I thought about the weak tweet I'd inevitably respond with, the kind of thing I always said when she said something crazy. "I love my mother very much but . . ." Or "family is wonderful because we can disagree and still love each other. . . ."

Mom had been to Israel on book tours, but I'd never been there. We weren't those kinds of Jews. Maybe my mom *had* thought of herself as that kind of Jew, but we had never been Israel Jews. Our family had come over in the 1800s during the Ukrainian pogroms and all my grandparents had been born in this country, except my grandmother who was born in London. We were the kind of Jews who didn't think of ourselves as "all that Jewish." We were the kind of Jews who passed, but still believed that people who weren't Jewish were just the tiniest bit antisemitic.

After about twenty minutes, my son came in and announced it was time to go. I was thrilled. I realized I'd forgotten to ask my mother about Martha Updike. Would she even be able to answer? Would she even know that Martha had, most assuredly, died? Did my mother even know where *she* was? Did she still know her own name? But maybe it was better that way, because if she did know, then there was a strong chance that she would get into the whole "You put us in a home to die!" discourse. Recently, Ken had roused himself from his deathbed to suggest that we make the "little apartment" (their rooms in the nursing home, in other words) my office when they moved back home.

I still hadn't told them we'd sold their apartment.

12

On November 2, 2023, I celebrated twenty-six years of sobriety. And then on the next day, I went back to the apartment on Sixty-Ninth Street. I went to sort through things. The apartment was about to no longer be mine. But there was still stuff there. Paintings by my grandmother. Paintings by my lesbian aunt who died alone in the Hebrew Home for the Aged in Riverdale, the aunt who forgot she was gay. Or that's what my mom said. Who knew what was true anymore. I was just so tired.

I'd gotten up early to practice my religion, the one thing that made me feel really truly good: being on television. I had gotten up at 4:45 a.m. and had gone to a TV studio in a hired car. Then I came home to take the children to school. Then I went to the apartment, the one I had grown up in.

We paid a woman to help me sort through all the stuff. There was always a woman, some woman, any woman, we paid to help us do things for us. Had this woman not been there, I don't know what I would have done. Maybe nothing. Maybe I would have just left everything and begged the people who were buying the apartment to throw everything out.

There were closets and closets filled with her clothes from the seventies, eighties, and nineties. She loved loud, wildly inappropriate clothing and gravitated toward shades of red. I pulled out some dresses from the closet: Gucci, Etro, Versace, and Dolce & Gabbana. I would never wear Dolce because the designers said horrible things about gay marriage and race, but Mom didn't remember that, or just was able to remove herself from it. I knew the pieces in her closet really well. I knew when they had been purchased, and if they'd been bought at their full retail price or on sale. I had been with her when she bought these clothes at Bergdorf Goodman, where she loved to go, either to check out or to feel better.

My mother truly believed that almost all problems could be solved (or at the very least addressed) with a trip to Bergdorf's. My mother, my brilliant, studious, serious mother, a woman who never got a grade below a B, loved to shop, specifically at Bergdorf Goodman. She inherited this obsession from her mother, who also believed all problems could be solved if you looked polished—and rich—enough. There was always a feeling in the family that a new dress, a good new winter coat, perhaps a fur (sorry), or a gorgeous new handbag from Bergdorf's could solve all your problems. Things could or would be okay if only you looked as if things were okay. My mother felt that dressing me beautifully was her job. The other parts of parenting she was not as interested in, but dressing me, *that* was her job.

"Should we go to *Bergdorf's?*" she would say.

My palms would get all hot and sweaty whenever she'd suggest this. Bergdorf Goodman with her was always a grand expedition, and I felt that anything could happen with her there, anything was possible. Bergdorf Goodman was a fantasy space and there was always a feeling of limitless possibility there; the right dress would solve all my problems, the right coat would get me that job or that boyfriend or that book deal. Shopping led to clothing and clothing led to magic.

We'd fly into the lobby of that magnificent limestone palace on Fifty-Eighth Street, and we'd stay for hours and hours. We wouldn't simply *try on* tops or skirts like normal people. We'd go, floor by floor, gathering up endless pieces of clothing in our arms, the more beautiful and the more expensive the better, then, in a flurry, we'd try on our bounty. The times when I was "fat," nothing would fit; when I was "thin," everything looked fantastic. Mom would make me add up the total cost of everything I wanted to buy. (I couldn't do math, can't do math, not even a little bit at all, so the figure I'd get would always be wrong.) She'd have everything shipped back to our house in Connecticut to save the sales tax.

When we'd arrive at the house on Fridays, she'd hide all Bergdorf Goodman boxes so Ken wouldn't see them. On Sundays when we drove back to the city, she'd have to get all the stuff out to the car also without Ken seeing. We absolutely could not afford any of the gorgeous things she bought herself and me. Like a night spent doing cocaine and Jägermeister shots, the next day would always be filled with remorse. A truth in life: the bill always comes due. And when my mom's quite literal bill (in the form of an AmEx statement) would arrive, Ken would reliably blow his top. The whole thing felt like waking up with a bad hangover as you tried to remember what had happened, the night before. From a very young age, I understood that shopping was as much of a drug as real drugs were, and I loved the experience of getting wasted at Bergdorf's with my mom.

So. I saved a few of my mom's favorite Gucci dresses and sold the rest.

I emptied out the storage units in Connecticut, too. Just stacks and stacks of paintings of my mom, photos of my mom, and pictures of my mom. She was on the cover of magazines and inside newspapers. She saved everything with her picture on it. I couldn't even feel anything. I didn't cry. I just told the woman to give most of the stuff to Housing Works. Maybe someone out there wants old pictures of Erica Jong.

My cousin Maria is a real estate agent and she had sold the apartment. When I was looking at a huge painting of my mother, Maria called me, but I declined the call. I couldn't talk. I didn't want to cry. Ken had had the portrait painted for her. It was very tacky, just the kind of thing my mother loved: in it she was rendered a blurry figure floating over Venice. Who has portraits painted of themselves? Erica Jong did. I stared at this stupid painting, feeling that it was confronting me to take some kind of action. But I couldn't take any action. I looked at that blond woman airborne over Venice—that illusive, elusive figure, that person who always left me waiting. I would look in the window of every passing taxi, wondering if she was inside. She never was.

I'd built this whole thing on a lie. This whole childhood, waiting for this woman to come home, to come to me, and she was never even there. She was floating above it all.

There were also paintings of me. I kept those. There were photos and watercolors by Henry Miller. Saved those, too. There were posters from rooms in the house in Weston. There was paper. Mom had saved notebooks. Mom had saved everything.

Her archive was at Columbia, but the rest of the contents of her life were handed to Housing Works. We weren't taking apart an apartment: we were disassembling the great Erica Jong. We were dismantling her. Soon the stuff would be gone. Soon

Mom would be gone. Soon this would be over. All the pain she caused me, all the pain I caused her—that would remain, but the rest would turn into dust.

I also finally sold their book collection. Was it worst thing I'd ever done? Probably. Definitely. And I didn't even hesitate. Just sold the whole collection the first chance I got. I told myself it was because books don't store well. I told myself it was because the paper disintegrates in your fingers. I told myself that books aren't stable. I told myself all the lies we tell ourselves. I got rid of the books because I was jealous of the weird codependent life my mother and stepdad had together. We tell ourselves stories so that we may live, to quote Joan Didion, a serious writer who never took Mom seriously. The truth was something slightly more sinister, the truth was a bitter mélange of jealousy and expectation. The truth was: I wanted their happiness to go away. You never grow out of your unhappy childhood. You are never *not* that unhappy bitter little girl; even now, even at forty-five, I'm still the sad, angry girl who is the last-picked for sports, the last-invited to sleepovers, forever waiting for my mom to show up at a school event—*any* school event. And she never shows up. She never comes, not once.

The apartment was gone, the books were gone. No more chances to pretend I was thirteen again. There was no more pretend. I was a grown-up now. I could never move home because . . .

Home was gone.

***

I got the text from my mother's aide when I was sitting down on my sofa with *The New York Times Book Review*. Mom was on the cover. It was the fiftieth anniversary of *Fear of Flying*. We knew we'd get some press for it, but no one thought it would be on the cover. Johnny was one of those aides who is overinvolved in a good way, kind of obsessive, and thank God for him. I needed someone to care. I cared, but I was also super busy and super depressed. Between the husband and the mother stuff, I would lie in bed and weep silently three or four nights a week.

"You need to call your mother," Johnny texted. "She must take a shower."

Great. Amazing. I would have to take this up with the woman herself. I packed the *TBR* into my bag and took myself down Lexington Avenue—my preferred route—to the nursing home. It was a few days before Thanksgiving and it was almost dark now, at 4:00 p.m. It was warm and gray. I punched her number in my phone.

"Hello, darling," she said. She was still so grand, but now in an odd, diminished sort of way.

"Mom," I said, "you need to take a shower."

"I'm drinking *coffee*, darling."

"I *know*, Mom," I replied, "but I *really* need you to go take a shower. The lady is there to help you."

"But I'm just waking up," she said.

It was 11:00 a.m. I had been up since 5:00 a.m., but of course it wasn't a contest. I had to go out and *do* things, while she was just running out the clock, trying to burn off the rest of her life. Since January, I had been living in a washing machine of Husband's Cancer and Mother's Dementia. Ken's Parkinson's-related dementia had now devolved to the point that he was in the hospital. He had a full-time aide and I hadn't visited him. I had wanted to, maybe? No, I don't really think I had wanted to. But Matt was going in the hospital for a minor scar-revision thing, and I had decided I could only do Hospital for husband on this particular day. All of this on the day Mom was on the cover of *The New York Times Book Review*.

I had never seen the photo they used for the cover. Were there tons of photos of Young Mom that I'd never encountered? Her chronic exhibitionism had made me slightly terrified of what was lurking out there. What if I happened upon a naked portrait? No, wait, I'd already seen that one: sitting in my storage facility in Long Island.

My whole life my mother had complained about her books rarely being reviewed in the *TBR* (this was not actually true) and now here she was on the cover. She'd always felt that she wasn't taken seriously by the literary community, such as it was. This was all happening too late. She was finally getting the deep and scholarly critical (although maybe a little mean) appraisal she'd always desired, and she didn't understand any of it.

It was a smart piece, but it still made Mom sound sort of small. Though it was very meaningful, just by the fact that it was published at all. In an attention economy nothing is more meaningful than attention, of course.

I came into her apartment, waving the *New York Times Book Review*. I had brought my little dog Bu with me.

"But they didn't even call me," she said.

She looked deflated. She was sitting in the little front room, at a white table. We were surrounded by paintings that my grandparents had painted. She was wearing an old shirt. I regret to report that she again wasn't wearing a bra. I tried not to get too close to her. I didn't want to know if she smelled. Later, I would complain that they weren't bathing her. I would call them and text the head of memory care. The thing that I hated most about visiting was the smell. The people who cleaned the place used a pine-smelling spray on the wall-to-wall carpet. It smelled like a horrible forest in a horrible land made of plastic and filled with plastic trees.

"That's irrelevant," I said. And then I had to ask the question. "Why *would The New York Times* have called you?"

She didn't have an answer for that.

"I didn't even know it was happening," she sullenly reiterated.

Why couldn't she have been happy about this? She had finally gotten what she'd wanted, but now it was meaningless. Did she even understand what any of it meant? Did she even remember that she had a legacy? And does a legacy even matter if you don't remember what you'd done and who you were?

"They didn't even try and get me on the phone," she added for good measure.

The great tragedy here was that all Mom had ever wanted was to matter as much as the men did. She'd always wanted to have the legacy of Philip Roth or John Updike . . . but now no one remembered them either. Maybe it wasn't that *women* writers didn't matter, maybe it was that *writers* in general no longer mattered. Could it really have been that everything she'd worked so hard for didn't exist anymore? It wasn't just that book coverage in magazines was relegated to the "book page" (this used to be the old complaint), it was now that there *was* no book page (and there were no magazines), and that books were important only insofar as they were able to get the momentary attention of a movie star who might include them in their book club.

Imagine that everything you've spent your entire life believing in was no longer true. Mom was now like the factory worker when the plant closed down. But it was almost worse than that: what she made was no longer valued, the plant closed down because no one valued what she, or any of us, made. She made widgets and people didn't want widgets anymore. They wanted short videos of people talking about celebrities, they wanted threads, they wanted free content. Oh, but that was wrong, too. Who even knew what the people wanted? But one of the things we *did* know was that people didn't want long meditations on life in the seventies for affluent white women. And sexism was no longer the central idea people cared about; it was just one of many, many factors.

Here is the first paragraph from the piece, by Jane Kamensky:

"Fifty years ago last month, Erica Jong published a debut novel that went on to sell more than 20 million copies. 'Fear of Flying,' a book so sexually frank that you may have found it hidden in your mother's underwear drawer, broke new ground in the explicitness of writing by and for women. Jong's heroine, Isadora Wing, was a live wire. She was also a dead end, certainly for Jong, and maybe for feminism, too."

Was it all a dead end?

The *TBR* piece continued with little digs, but I hesitate to get stuck on them because honestly just being in *The New York Times* these days is more meaningful than what *The New York Times* says about you. Also, I would add, my mother has always been her own worst enemy, and she made herself small by being so narcissistic. Had she been able to pull back and see herself as a piece of a larger puzzle, that would have changed everything for her, and for me, and for all of us feminists.

In 1977, a year before I was born, there was a review of my mother's book *How to Save Your Own Life* in the *TBR*. It's by the late, great critic John Leonard, and he hit on something important, something I'd felt my whole life. From the piece:

"It's probably none of my business, but I wonder whether the private person got lost on the lecture circuit between talk shows, where she was forever reading aloud the poems she had written while working on 'Fear of Flying,' and the letters she had received about 'Fear of Flying,' and the poems she had written about the letters she had received and her feelings on finishing 'Fear of Flying.' As she told Mademoiselle last June, 'I'm one of the most interviewed people in the world.' Being interviewed demands very little from a celebrity—much less a myth—but time and canned opinions. It is as if, in 'How to Save Your Own Life,' Erica Jong had interviewed herself, when she should have been, sentence by sentence, writing a book. Sincerity is no excuse for sloppy craft."

That was it. John Leonard got it. There was no version of Mom who was just for me. There was only one Erica Jong and that Erica Jong was the same one who spoke at classes and on *Donahue*. Her fans got the same Erica Jong I did. There was no private individual. There was just Erica Jong, Feminist Icon, except that she was really not that feminist, and really not that iconic.

Now, during what should have been her moment of triumph, she looked so small and defeated. I made her pose for a picture, holding the *Book Review* up to her face. It felt as if I were taking a proof-of-life photo. I knew the picture was in slightly poor taste, but I had to do it. I wondered if I should post the photo of my mom, but her face... there was something very *wrong* with her face. She didn't have her same face anymore. It was hard to explain, but there was something profoundly off about her eyes. She had the same blue eyes, light blue, kind of milky almost, but there was something wrong about them. Like a picture missing an element. She didn't look like herself anymore. She had that look in her eyes, that blank look the crazy guy in my AA meeting had, the guy who was almost handsome if you squinted, but if you looked closely you could see that he was just the slightest bit not right.

I had to remind myself: she wasn't dead, she was on this planet still, sort of. She was my mother. She was still the great Erica Jong.

Well, *ish*.

13

Ken died on December 14. A few days after he left the hospital, the nursing home told me it was time for hospice care. They set up hospice in their apartment at the nursing home. I called the doctor, another fancy, expensive doctor, and he told me that Ken's heart no longer worked and that that was why his lungs kept filling up with fluid. Howard Fast died that way, too. He drowned. The doctor told me it was past time for hospice care. I didn't want to fight with the doctors, also I needed to think of myself as someone who could say goodbye when it was time. I think of myself as a person who isn't sentimental, someone who is rational. (I am not that way, not even a little, but we all have our delusions.)

The hospice people came to see Ken. They got him undressed and looked at his skin. I couldn't tell if he could understand what was happening. There was something so horrible about seeing him, just for a second, with no shirt, looking so lost. Johnny the aide was helping him. I wanted to die.

I signed all the forms. I knew it was a big deal because the forms were on a tablet like an iPad, but a kind of heavy-duty one. As I signed the forms, I thought about Jimmy Carter, who'd been in hospice for months and months. Hospice can last for months,

I think to myself. Years, even. Besides it's December, and right before Christmas. Ken can't die on Christmas.

And then he died.

The whole thing took like three days. The hospice people gave him morphine. My cousin said his brother wanted to come by, so could they keep him alive until then? This made me furious, but I didn't say anything. Almost immediately, Ken seemed to be unconscious, in a state of dying that looked like a coma. I came in and out of the room, like a visitor. I didn't stay for hours like I should have. I couldn't face it.

This is not one of those stories where the daughter nurses her parents. I am the daughter who finds people and pays them to do the daughterly work that I might have done had I been a good daughter.

I spend a lot of time wondering if I'm not taking care of them because they didn't take care of me. I spend a lot of time wondering if I hadn't been raised by nannies would I be a better daughter. Is this my way of getting them back for that unhappy childhood I find myself unable to escape? Am I trying to get back at them? Am I, at twenty-six years sober, finally trying to settle the score?

At one point, Ken's hair was all slicked down and it looked as if he were using his entire body to breathe. I could smell the minty pine stuff they used on the carpets: it burned my nostrils. Everything was burning itself into my brain. These were the memories I didn't want. But these are memories I will have.

I found my mom wandering around in the hall. She was lost.

"He's going to be okay, right?" she asked me.

"No, Mom," I said. "He is not going to be all right."

"But he *might* be?"

"No," I said.

She considered this for a moment.

"Maybe I'll get remarried then."

"Maybe," I said. I hugged her. "Maybe you should."

I ran out to do TV. I did it because I needed to work, because work made me feel good and because everything else made me feel bad. I did TV right after I watched the hospice-ambulance people give my stepfather a dose of morphine from a weird plastic container that was sealed and connected with some weird plastic ties, though it wasn't really an ambulance, because they weren't there to save the patient.

Later I will wonder if hospice had maybe given him too much morphine. Now I know how Matt felt when his father died.

My stepsister—who is not really my stepsister, because Ken didn't have kids, but is the daughter of one of his ex-girlfriends—looked at Ken and said, "Is he supposed to sleep like that?"

I have no idea what dying is supposed to look like, but I suspected that she was right in her supposition that something was terribly wrong with the way Ken was dying. I'd watched my friend Samantha Stein fight to breathe those last few days when we kept a vigil at her bedside. Sometimes the fight to survive comes down only to the struggle to breathe.

I left. I'm always leaving now. I always have somewhere I must go. Often, I'm just running somewhere—running *away* as much as running *to*. I pay someone to sit with my mother. Just like she paid someone to watch me. Matt was furious with me because I'd spent all the cash in our bank account—not only on my mom, but also on things like Ubers, and dinners, and expensive black T-shirts, and vet bills. Is the money I spend to have someone sit with my mom the most frivolous use of our money, or is it the least frivolous? There is something deeply weird about paying this woman, who is literally named Comfort, to be my mother's daughter so I don't have to. I know the whole thing is weird and wrong, but I also don't want to sit with my mother.

At 5:30 a.m. on the day Ken died, I woke up to missed calls from the aide, from the nurse, from the nursing home. I started calling all those missed numbers. I learned that he just didn't wake up; he just stopped breathing. Mom slept through it all. She was in the bed next to him, but she slept through it. We are good sleepers but bad wives. A good wife wouldn't have slept through her husband's death, but a good daughter wouldn't have gone home to watch TV. Sleeping through Ken's death is as good a metaphor as any for all the stuff I've missed.

Now I'm the head of this weird, fractured family which consists of just my mother and me. I decided to get the funeral done right away. I wanted it over with. I begged the funeral home to do the funeral the following day; this was an insane request, but I didn't care. I just needed it to be over. Jews tend to get the funeral done quickly. It was a Thursday, and the next day was (obviously) Friday, then was Saturday, and you're not supposed to do stuff on Saturday because of the Sabbath.

I realized that I was supposed to say something about Ken at the funeral.

I wrote down two things on a piece of paper: one of them was about their small plane and the other was about the sailboat they had—big, forty-eight feet, no crew. "Your *mom* is the crew," he'd tell me. I went on that boat twice. Once it caught fire. The coast guard knew them because they'd had so many incidents. I was not sure why I thought this was appropriate to talk about at a funeral.

Ken's brother wanted to say some words. I let him. Ken's sister had died four months before, so Ken's brother was now a pro at eulogies. They were a story by Edgar Allan Poe; they were the House of Usher. I'd recently watched the series *The Fall of the House of Usher* on Netflix. All the children die in rapid succession because the father made a deal with the Devil for money. Everyone falls like dominoes, one death leads to the next, then the next, then the next. Apparently, the family in *The Fall of the House of Usher* is based not so much on the Poe story, but on the Sacklers, the owners of Purdue Pharma, the company that created OxyContin and ruined America. Except I knew the Sacklers and they weren't like the people in the movie. (Or the characters in the Poe story.) Also, the Sackler we knew died, and the rest of the family fled the country (which does seem kind of crime-y).

Anyway. I knew that when I got up there, I was either going to be okay, or not. And I wasn't sure it mattered. I kept coming back to how thin the line is between normal and completely falling apart. I kept thinking about this horrible year, this midlife-crisis year. I kept wondering when all this would end.

Or maybe it never ends, maybe everyone keeps dying until there's no one left, *Usher*-style.

My mother's assistant, who I guess is my assistant now, too—I finally have an assistant though she's not entirely mine (which is in some ways peak nepo)—sent me this text:

"The night aide says your mom woke up three times and sat up and talked to her about Ken. Every time the aide gently told her it was important to go to sleep because she had a big day coming up."

A big day. A big day for Erica Jong used to be being on television, or giving a speech, or accepting an award, but now my mother no longer does things like that, so her big day is burying her husband.

My college kid is traveling back from school to attend the funeral, but he lost his wallet and then he had to beg TSA to let him on the flight to New York. I sent pictures of his passport. He eventually talked his way onto the flight. I was both furious and oddly not. I was in that weird haze of grief. I went to Starbucks twice. I ate a bag of cough drops. I watched TV.

Before the funeral, I went to an AA meeting. I wore pink sneakers. I felt a wave of grief. I shared at the meeting, one of those shares that's designed to make people feel badly for you. In AA, we talk a lot about being "of service" and I try to end conversations in meetings with an offer to "be helpful." As in "How can I be helpful to you?" And although I felt like an actress in the meeting, I wanted to be helpful to the people there, I really did.

I walked from my AA meeting to the funeral home, Frank Campbell, on Madison Avenue. It's a very fancy funeral home, Frank Campbell, super expensive, but I wasn't sure you could negotiate on the cost of a funeral. Growing up, I had always wanted to attend a funeral there (is that a weird thing to say?), but the place wasn't considered Jewish. Jewish funerals happened on the West Side, at that depressing place on Riverside. But I thought, *fuck it*, we'll have it near my house.

Frank Campbell is pretty, and clean, and doesn't smell like lilies. I hate lilies. They smell like death. There were a lot of people there, many I knew from growing up, and lots of my mom and stepfather's friends. The rabbi who married Matt and me got up to speak.

Mom sat nervously in the front row. Her head kept bobbing. She now has some kind of neurological thing that makes her head bob back and forth like a chicken pecking seeds. I know that's a mean thing to say. Ken's brother spoke. Ken's other stepdaughter spoke. Then Mom looked over at me and whispered, "They're going to want me to say something, right?"

Oh God. I feel a chill. *She wants to say something.* I should have known she would want to say something. She has never *not* wanted to say something. This was a woman who spoke at everything—weddings she was barely invited to, parties she wandered by. Sometimes she was pretty good, though. I will give her that.

I was reminded about a story Dad had once told me about my mom giving a speech at her grandfather's funeral. My mom was obsessed with Papa Mirsky, as they called him. He was a Russian Jew, and a portrait painter. He was her person. He lived to the ripe old age of one hundred and four. Not that the later years were so golden, though—she once told me that he begged her to kill him. "It's just too *long*," he said. They were sitting on our porch in Weston, staring out at the trees. Everyone he knew was dead. "Why does God want to punish me by keeping me on this planet forever?" he asked.

Mom refused to kill him.

Dad had told me that she had eulogized him for way too long, about forty-five minutes, and then at some point she'd gone into a whole thing about how he would burn in hell.

"*Burn in hell?*" I had asked my dad on the phone.

"Burn in hell."

"But Jews don't believe in hell," I had said. "And Mom loved Papa in a way she didn't love her parents. Or, really, anyone."

That included me.

"Why did she say that, Dad?"

"I honestly don't know." He paused. "I really couldn't tell you."

Would she say that Ken was also going to burn in hell?

In this moment, I realized that I couldn't say no to her. I couldn't say no to my mom. I couldn't tell her she was not permitted to speak at her husband's funeral. Of course I couldn't do that, even though there was a distinct possibility that this could all go very, very wrong. My glamorous mom with whom I had always been so totally, completely, utterly obsessed, but was now avoiding like the plague. My chic mom who used to be smart but who now had a head filled with sawdust.

I relented.

"Sure," I said.

But I know that I would have to go up there with her. Then at least if I needed to pry her off the stage, I could do it quickly.

We went up together. We stood at the small podium. It felt unstable. I feel this might be a metaphor.

"Where is the microphone?" she asked, searching around. Once a performer always a performer.

There was no microphone, but one was not needed—we weren't speaking to a football stadium. I looked out at the room of people, many of whom I'd known my whole life. Ken was eighty-two. He was old, but not exceptionally old. His death was sad, but not tragic. This was not one of those funerals where people wondered what happened. Everyone there knew that Ken had been in and out of dementia for a while, they knew that he was sometimes in his body and sometimes in some otherworldly plane.

"Ken was the kindest man," my mother said, and paused. She didn't have her usual bravado anymore, that crazy energy and charisma she had when I was young. "I loved him so much. He took such good care of me."

It wasn't a brilliant talk, but it was coherent, and it was very much from the heart. The kind of speech a person gives about her husband after thirty years of marriage.

As she spoke, it occurred to me that she must have really loved Ken a lot.

Now it was my turn. I worried that my eulogy wouldn't be as heartfelt as my mother's. I ended up telling a story about Ken and the airplane, and once when he was flying it, the window opened and his wallet got sucked out. I also told the story of the first time he met my grandma—my mother's mother—and I explained that because she (my grandmother) was such an impossible person, he decided to stay with Mom. Mom needed him. Ken went where he was needed.

As I spoke, I realized, perhaps for the first time, that he was a wonderful man, and a wonderful stepfather. And that the problem—my constant disapproval, my judgmental nature—had always been mine. My fucking problem. The problem was *me*, not him. Not *them*. I had been a bad stepdaughter. I had been mean and cranky, I realized as I spoke, and I understood, finally, and too late, that Ken had deserved better than me. I should have been there in the hospital, every hour, every minute. I should have slept by his bed. I could have and should have done more. I was a bad stepdaughter. And a bad daughter.

The worst daughter, actually.

After I finished my eulogy, I sat down next to my mom. My small mom. My diminished mom. I took her hand. She looked at me, expectant.

"I guess they're going to want me to speak now," she said.

HOW TO LOSE YOUR MOTHER

"No, Mom. You just spoke."

"Oh, I did?"

"Yes, Mom."

"Was I any good?"

"Yes," I said. "You were."

***

Later, we sat shiva again at my apartment. My apartment, which I've lived in for sixteen years. It was one of those weird Fridays in December: too warm, too dark. People ate. I wished I still smoked. Eventually everyone went home. I lay on the sofa and watched TV with my teenage sons. I thought about texting my father-in-law to tell him about the evening, but he was dead, too.

We had just sat shiva for my father-in-law, and my stepfather's sister. We kept burying family members. I wondered if eventually there would be no one left to bury. Eventually we'd run out of people, right?

We put out huge spreads of food, lots of bagels and cream cheese. We had cupcakes. We had all sorts of cheese. I lingered over the food. I love to check out with food. I love to check out period. Part of being an alcoholic is loving to check out.

During the shiva it was again unclear that my mother understood that Ken was dead. People asked me this question a lot, and I answered it as I answer so many questions now: "I don't know." And I really *don't* know. I don't know what sticks in her weird brain now and I don't know what's real to her and what's not real, and I don't know what's happening in there anymore, and maybe I never did.

***

After Ken died, we went to California. I left my mom in New York. When I was packing, I kept thinking about Joan Didion's famous quote about the state:

> California is a place in which a boom mentality and a sense of Chekhovian loss meet in uneasy suspension; in which the mind is troubled by some buried but ineradicable suspicion that things better work here, because here, beneath the immense bleached sky, is where we run out of continent.

I knew I was being a bad daughter, leaving my mother alone on Christmas, and the knowledge that she'd been a bad mother did not make me feel better this time.

Matt, the kids, and I flew out early in the morning. On the flight to L.A., I kept thinking about Mom sitting alone in those two little rooms, watching television, drinking wine. I also thought about how proud I was of myself to have, pretty much, conquered my fear-ish of flying. I still obsessed before I flew, but when I was finally on the plane, I was mostly fine. I didn't pray on this flight. I didn't cross myself. I didn't convince myself that the sound of the landing gear was proof that something had gone horrifically wrong and that we were all going to die. I didn't fantasize about Valium. I was proud that I wasn't that girl anymore. I am sober and sort of sane and not my mother. And, yes, I understand that there is something so pathetic about being forty-five and congratulating myself for not overdosing on Valium during a flight, but these alcoholic instincts are thick ridges and are hard to smooth. You don't become unalcoholic; you're always alcoholic, you just learn not to drink.

HOW TO LOSE YOUR MOTHER

"Another holiday of being a bad daughter," I told Matt on the flight.

"Dr. Makari has a theory about this," he replied.

Matt had been seeing his therapist Dr. Makari since before we met. Dr. Makari had a theory about how the children of alcoholics try to become the parents they never had, at least I think that's what it was. But Matt never knew what it was like to be the child of an alcoholic. He truly loved his unalcoholic parents, so much so that he even thought his mother was a wonderful cook. She was a terrible cook.

I was sad about Ken, but it was hard to feel too sad when we landed in L.A. The sun was bright and there was a feeling that everything would, theoretically, be okay here. Los Angeles is a place where possibilities are endless. L.A. is good. L.A. can reset your life. My parents thought L.A. would make me a drug addict, but I became a drug addict on my own, without L.A.'s help. L.A. had always been good to me.

I thought about Bret Easton Ellis when we drove from LAX; it was impossible not to. As we left the airport in a rental car, I remembered this passage from *Less Than Zero*: "People are afraid to merge on freeways in Los Angeles. This is the first thing I hear when I come back to the city. Blair picks me up from LAX and mutters this under her breath as she drives up the onramp. She says, 'People are afraid to merge on freeways in Los Angeles.' Though that sentence shouldn't bother me, it stays in my mind for an uncomfortably long time. Nothing else seems to matter."

For some reason, I believed it would be a good idea to stay at Shutters in Santa Monica, but I forgot that, as much as I love L.A., I hate Santa Monica. But Santa Monica and Shutters made Matt happy, and Matt had cancer. It was too cold for the beach and the tide was scary and people kept getting swept up in it. There was something kind of poetic and odd about the tide sweeping people up.

We drove to Palm Springs, to visit my father. It took about two hours to get there and we passed lots of wind turbines. We got a meal at an In-N-Out Burger. (Four dollars.) Outside the restaurant, there was that odd agricultural smell, which is, to me, the smell of Southern California. My thoughts went back to Joan Didion again. Can't go to California, can't write about California, without thinking about Didion. Didion owns the state and always will.

I arrived at my dad's house in the early afternoon. He lives in a golf development, although he does not play golf. My dad and stepmom came out to the car and held me in their arms. We kept holding on to each other that way for a very long time.

I had spent so much time thinking about the demise of my parents, but there was a set of parents right here, waiting for me.

I wept that night—not in front of them, but in the shower, my safe space for crying. I cried and repeated these words to myself over and over again: *My parents were here this whole time.*

The trip to California was six times as expensive as Matt thought it had been. I put the whole bill on my AmEx without telling Matt the actual sum and decided I'd figure out a way to pay for it eventually. (I am, in my financial irresponsibility, exactly like my mother.) On January 3, when we were back in the city, Matt had a scan at Sloan Kettering—a scan of his bones and lungs and liver to see if the cancer had spread there. We were most worried about the bones. When cancer goes to the bones, that's when it's bad, very bad.

I offered to go with him. He declined. I didn't push.

The next day, I forced him to check the results on the portal.

"I don't want to," he said.

"You have to."

He acquiesced. "No evidence of metastasis," he read. The margins were clean. The liver was clean. The lungs were clean. The bones, they were clean, too. Everything was clean.

The following morning, we went to Dr. O'Reilly's office. We decided to walk. It was one of those unnaturally warm January days, and the sky was cloudless and so profoundly blue. It was just pure blue ocean reflection.

Matt stopped walking. He bent down to tie his shoes, which irritated me for some vague reason. And then, suddenly, it was as if we were back to being normal people in a normal marriage. We were starting to annoy each other again, like normal married people.

We put on masks in the lobby of Sloan Kettering. A maintenance guy told Matt that his mask was on inside out.

In the waiting room, a woman my age was saying something about tumors all over her body. "My doctor has a theory about my tumors," she told her people. They all nodded.

We were called into the waiting room a minute or two after that. Little blond Dr. O'Reilly had good news.

"As you saw on the portal, everything looks clean," she said. "You have clean margins; you have clean bones. The lungs look good."

There's always something odd, something strange, about good news; we never fully accept it, even when we do. And we'd seen the portal; I'd bullied Matt into checking it.

She said that he would have to keep taking the lanreotide

once a month, but that he wouldn't need a scan for another six months.

We walked home under that same blue sky.

I kept avoiding picking up Ken's ashes. I didn't want to. I couldn't go back to my year of death; I couldn't face it. The ashes would be the anvil that pulled me under forevermore. But I knew I had to get them. Ken's remains had nowhere else to go.

On January 17, I decided to return to the funeral home. I did *Morning Joe* and walked back uptown. It was very cold, so cold my face hurt. It was cold the way it used to be cold when I was young, before New York City got classified as subtropical. I was worried Frank Campbell might be closed, but the door opened right up for me. The woman working in the front had done Ken's funeral. She had a kindly-looking face, soft features. She was young, in her twenties or thirties.

"Remind me your name?" she asked, apologetic.

I told her that his name is—was—Ken Burrows. Then I told her my name.

She looked even more apologetic.

"I'm so sorry," she said. "But I need to see some ID."

I handed her my driver's license. I could imagine people being furious with her asking for their identification, but I absolutely knew it had to be some kind of New York State regulation and I could imagine that the fine for hiding the recipient when you release human remains could be in the tens of thousands of dollars. Maybe they could even lose their license if they gave "human remains" to the wrong person? Who knew.

But while I understood that she didn't want to give the wrong ashes to the wrong person, weren't the ashes all really the same when you got right down to it?

As I sat there in the lobby of the funeral home, I thought about those two words: *human remains*. These are the bits of the human that remain after the life and the memories and the flesh and the water and the stuff that rots are gone. This is the ash. The ash is permanent. The ash can be put on a bookshelf. The ash is what remains.

The lobby of the funeral parlor was cold. It was late enough in January that we'd given up on the concept of light and had just embraced the gray leafless trees. She took my driver's license and came back a few minutes later with a form on which a copy of my license was attached. I signed my name. Next to my name was a place to indicate what my relation was to him. I was going to write "stepdaughter," but I didn't.

Instead, I wrote "daughter."

As I walked home, carrying my stepdad's ashes, I called my dad, my actual dad. It was so cold I could barely feel my fingers.

I didn't tell him I love him. I didn't tell him that I wrote "daughter" on the form when I picked up Ken's ashes. I thought it would make him sad and I didn't want to make him sad.

I knew that I now had such a limited window with him, with my mom, with my stepmother, with all of them, and I didn't want to waste that. I didn't want to hurt them. I was a bad daughter, but I didn't have to be.

My mother had been a negligent parent, and it was impossible for her to be otherwise. She was a damaged person, and she wasn't a bad person. She tried her best. And it is true that sometimes your best is actually not good at all. Sometimes your best is *terrible*. The fact is that she did love me and gave me everything she had to give: it never felt like enough, but maybe it should have been? Maybe someday I'll be grateful for her, and for the life she tried to create for me. And now Ken was gone. The man had disappeared—the men always disappeared, eventually—and we were back where we started from. It was just the two of us, all over again.

When I got home, I put the bag on the sofa. I took out the urn. It was a square brown wood box. It looked like a book— same shape, same height and width. I knew all about books. I was an expert in books. For a while, I had a huge tower of books behind me in my home office where I appear on TV. I bought this urn because it looked like a book. Books are my life, and my family's.

I put Ken's urn on the shelf next to the urn of my sweet old dog Cerberus. My mom's opal ring shone on my finger in the remaining light of the day. "The good opals are dark," said the Sotheby's man with the British accent. I considered what it meant for a thing to be "good" and for a thing to be "bad." In this case, I assumed he meant that the light opals were more common than the dark ones. But I *was* dark, I was all darkness, and what I needed was light—common light. As tormented as she always was, and as fraught as our relationship could often be, my mother always found the light.

We started this annus horribilis 2023 with mothers and fathers (or in my case a stepfather). We started this annus horribilis with Matt having a full pancreas and a spleen and also a gallbladder. We started 2023 as middle-aged children with parents.

Sometime in 2023, between the hospitalizations and the shivas, and the talks with the rabbis and the conversations with nurses and aides, and my cable-news hits, Matt and I started walking the dogs together around the block at night, sometimes 9:00 p.m., sometimes 10:00. We put all three of them in their little coats. The hairless dog whines and tries to make it hard to put his coat on. The fancy-breeder dog has long hair that always gets caught in the zipper. Spartacus, our very, very old dog, has trouble keeping up with the other two, but he tries hard. We named him after my grandfather's most famous book. There has always been a little—or a lot—of Howard Fast in him. Spartacus is a fighter.

One very cold night in January (hadn't it been January for a year?), we did our little walk down Madison with the dogs.

"Our parents are all dead," I said.

"No, they're not," Matt said. "My mom is alive. And your mom is alive. So is your dad."

Oh right.

I guess it was impossible to argue with the fact that his mom and my mom actually *were* alive, just not in the way we'd like them to be. But we had to be grateful for what remained. And I knew that I hadn't been grateful enough for them, or for any of it.

Mom was no longer in the world the way the rest of us were. She occupied a different plane. She was warehoused on Second Avenue, in a very expensive nursing home, waiting to die, watching cable news with her aide, Johnny, or with any of the other aides who take such good care of her. The aides adore her. And I would go see her, next week, or the week after, and we would talk about how much she loved me, talk about how much she liked watching me on television, whatever else she could think of. A better daughter would not have left her alone after her husband died. A better daughter would have moved her into her building, but I wasn't that daughter. Did I wish I *were* that daughter?

Maybe? But the main thing was that I had survived being her child.

Sometimes you just have to put the life jacket on yourself first.

I considered everything we'd lost forever in the past year: my stepfather, my father-in law, my aunt, thirty percent of Matt's pancreas, his gallbladder, and spleen. All these losses. And we don't get to redo any of it. A year ago, when Matt first got diagnosed, I kept telling myself that the only way through was through. We used to say that to each other, Matt and I: the only way through is through. Backward is not possible. We can only go forward.

Leo saw a poodle crossing Madison and started barking like a lunatic. Bucephalus joined in. The little old white dog is very refined and remained calm.

"I guess we're the grown-ups now," I said.

"I'm a fifty-nine-year-old man," Matt replied. "I would fucking *hope* I'm a grown-up."

But *I* wasn't fifty-nine; I was forty-five. One of the hazards of being married to someone a decade and a half older is that you always consider yourself young, but I wasn't young either, not now, and especially not after the year I'd had. I was in the middle of my life. I was about to enter the second half of my life. The end part. Watching the parents die off, making it very clear that we were the next generation to go.

I had spent so much time thinking about how to get out of my bad childhood. I had spent so much time beating myself up for being stuck in it, but I could never dislodge myself. You don't end your bad childhood simply because you want to. You don't get to decide when any of it ends.

HOW TO LOSE YOUR MOTHER

So much of life isn't a choice. You get sick. Medicines sometimes don't work. Sometimes people you love grow tumors in their pancreases. Sometimes those tumors are the "good tumors" and sometimes they're not. Organs refuse to do what they're supposed to. Kidneys stop. Hearts stop. Brains malfunction. Sometimes your kids have crises. Sometimes people betray you. Sometimes you betray them.

Your parents die and sometimes you're even a little glad that they're not suffering anymore . . . or that *you're* not suffering anymore. Sometimes you actually kind of *want* them to die, because that's the only way *you'll* ever grow up. But sometimes you need them and sometimes they slip through your fingers when you need them most of all.

I was the boring stable one now. I'd spent my whole life petrified my mother would blow up my life, and hers, but that hadn't happened. That hadn't happened.

I picked up Spartacus, the old-timer. Matt looked at me. I looked at him. I had bags under my eyes now, but Matt didn't care. He loved me. And I loved him.

We entered the new year as the adults we had to be.

January 2024

Acknowledgments

Thank you to:

    Mom and Dad and Barbara and the brothers and spouses and their kids

    My kids

    Pilar Queen

    Adrienne Miller

    Andrea Schulz

    Michael Calderone

    Radhika Jones

    Susan Cheever

    Ginny Grenham

    Jesse Cannon

    Katie Phang

    George Hahn

    Katie Benner

    Nicolle Wallace

    Marci Klein

    Mika Brzezinski

    Joey Scarborough

    Joe Scarborough